Flaxseed

Physicians, scientists and savvy laypeople want *reliable* information on foods and supplements that might improve the outcome in chronic diseases that otherwise shorten our lives. These health conditions include type 2 diabetes, heart attacks, high blood pressure, chronic kidney disease and others. Incorporating flaxseed into one's diet can greatly improve outcomes in various health conditions. Thousands of peer-reviewed articles have been published documenting the clinical efficacy of flaxseed as a whole or its individual components and reveal the *mechanisms* by which those various components work.

Flaxseed: Evidence-Based Cardiovascular and Other Medicinal Benefits is an encyclopedic and definitive text describing the health benefits of this humble plant. The book features exquisite detail on the three major components of the plant that are responsible for most of the documented benefits, those components being omega-3 fatty acids and two compounds that increase endothelial production of nitric oxide, those compounds being the amino acid L-arginine, and cyanogenic glycosides.

Attention Readers: If you are not already familiar with the health benefits of omega-3 fatty acids and of the above-named nitric oxide donors, then this book opens a vast world of scientific discovery that one can immediately apply to improving health. This book calls attention to a wealth of journal articles providing practical information on consuming flaxseed and its overall health benefits. Enjoy!

Flaxseed

Evidence-Based Cardiovascular and Other Medicinal Benefits

Robert Fried, PhD
Richard M. Carlton, MD

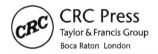

CRC Press is an imprint of the
Taylor & Francis Group, an **informa** business

First edition published 2023
by CRC Press
6000 Broken Sound Parkway NW, Suite 300, Boca Raton, FL 33487–2742

and by CRC Press
4 Park Square, Milton Park, Abingdon, Oxon, OX14 4RN

CRC Press is an imprint of Taylor & Francis Group, LLC

© 2023 Taylor & Francis Group, LLC

Reasonable efforts have been made to publish reliable data and information, but the author and publisher cannot assume responsibility for the validity of all materials or the consequences of their use. The authors and publishers have attempted to trace the copyright holders of all material reproduced in this publication and apologize to copyright holders if permission to publish in this form has not been obtained. If any copyright material has not been acknowledged please write and let us know so we may rectify in any future reprint.

Except as permitted under U.S. Copyright Law, no part of this book may be reprinted, reproduced, transmitted, or utilized in any form by any electronic, mechanical, or other means, now known or hereafter invented, including photocopying, microfilming, and recording, or in any information storage or retrieval system, without written permission from the publishers.

For permission to photocopy or use material electronically from this work, access www. copyright.com or contact the Copyright Clearance Center, Inc. (CCC), 222 Rosewood Drive, Danvers, MA 01923, 978-750-8400. For works that are not available on CCC please contact mpkbookspermissions@tandf.co.uk

Trademark notice: Product or corporate names may be trademarks or registered trademarks and are used only for identification and explanation without intent to infringe.

ISBN: 978-1-032-30274-4 (hbk)
ISBN: 978-1-032-30273-7 (pbk)
ISBN: 978-1-003-30428-9 (ebk)

DOI: 10.1201/b22986

Typeset in Times
by Apex CoVantage, LLC

Contents

Preface xi
Acknowledgments xiii
Disclaimer xv

Chapter 1 Introduction 1

    1.1   Flax—Garment of Pharaohs and Health-Giving Seeds 1
    1.2   Flax—A Functional Food 2
    1.3   Cyanogenic Glycosides (CNglcs) 3
    1.4   How Safe Is It to Consume Flaxseed? 3
    1.5   Disclaimer 6
          1.5.1   CAVEAT 7
    1.6   Supplement Dosages in Clinical and Research Trials 7
          1.6.1   Flaxseed 8
          1.6.2   Omega-3 PUFAs—Alpha-Linolenic Acid (ALA), Eicosapentaenoic Acid (EPA) and Docosahexaenoic Acid (DHA) 11
          1.6.3   L-Arginine 14
    1.7   Ad Lib Supplementation 18
          1.7.1   Raw Flaxseed 19
          1.7.2   Including Flaxseed in Daily Diet 21
    1.8   Summary 22
    1.9   References 22

Chapter 2 Flaxseed, a Functional Food—Constituents and Their Health Benefits 25

    2.1   Introduction 25
    2.2   Constituents That Make Flaxseed a Functional Food 25
    2.3   Flaxseed Oil/Lipid Components 26
    2.4   Proteins 27
    2.5   Dietary Fiber 28
    2.6   Lignans 29
    2.7   Minerals 29
    2.8   The Health Benefits of Flaxseed 29
    2.9   CNglcs in Flaxseeds, NO-Donors 34
    2.10 Guidelines to Supplementation of Flaxseed and Flaxseed Oil 35
          2.10.1 Recommended Flaxseed Supplement Content of ALA 37

	2.11	Potential Anti-Nutritional Aspects of Flaxseed 37
	2.12	Health Benefits of Flax Proteins.. 38
	2.13	Summary 39
	2.14	References... 39

Chapter 3 The Beneficial Effect of Omega-3 PUFA and L-Arginine on Endothelial Nitric Oxide (NO) Bioavailability 45

	3.1	The More You NO 45
	3.2	Nitric Oxide: The 1992 *Science* "Molecule of the Year" 46
	3.3	Bottom Line . . . the Endothelium 47
		3.3.1 The Structure and Function of the *Endothelium* 47
	3.4	How Does the Body Form NO?... 49
		3.4.1 Footnote to History... 49
	3.5	Reactive Oxygen Species (ROS) and Oxidative Stress—A Major Cause of Endothelium Damage.................. 50
	3.6	Endothelial NO from L-Arginine—Nitric Oxide Synthase (eNOS)... 51
	3.7	How Endothelium-Derived Nitric Oxide (eNO) Is Formed... 52
	3.8	NO Formed from CNglcs 53
	3.9	The Blood Vessels of the Blood Vessels (*Vasa Vasorum*) Are Regulated by NO 54
		3.9.1 Structure and Function of *Vasa Vasorum* 55
		3.9.2 Vasa Vasorum Depends Exclusively on Endothelium-Derived (NO) Vasorelaxation 56
	3.10	The Endothelial Glycocalyx 56
		3.10.1 The Glycocalyx Regulates eNO Formation................ 58
	3.11	The Endothelial Glycocalyx in Health and Disease................ 59
		3.11.1 Diabetes 59
		3.11.2 Atherosclerosis 60
		3.11.3 Hypertension... 60
		3.11.4 Kidney Function 61
	3.12	Summary 61
	3.13	References... 62

Chapter 4 The Role of Flaxseed Micronutrients and Nitric Oxide (NO) in Blood Vessel and Heart Function 67

	4.1	Introduction 67
	4.2	What Propels Blood through the Circulatory System? 68
		4.2.1 Systole.. 68
		4.2.2 Flaxseed Increases NO Bioavailability 70
		4.2.3 Flaxseed Omega-3 Fatty Acid, Alpha-Linolenic Acid, Promotes eNO Formation 70

		4.2.4 Flaxseed Improves the Ejection Fraction 71

	4.3	Arterial Vessel Compliance 72
		4.3.1 Flaxseed Oil Promotes Arterial Blood Vessel Elasticity (Compliance) 73
	4.4	The Arterial Waveform 74
	4.5	Measuring Blood Flow by Flow-Mediated Dilation (FMD) 76
		4.5.1 Flaxseed and L-Arginine Improve FMD 77
	4.6	Endothelial Nitric Oxide (eNO) and Control of Blood Pressure 79
		4.6.1 Endothelium-Independent Control of Blood Pressure 79
		4.6.2 Endothelium-Dependent Control of Blood Pressure 79
		4.6.3 Interaction of Endothelium-Independent and Endothelium-Dependent Blood Flow Control Systems 80
		4.6.4 The Role of NO in Vascular Remodeling in Hypertension 80
		4.6.5 Flaxseed Combats Hypertension 82
	4.7	Flaxseed Combats Peripheral Artery Disease (PAD) 83
	4.8	Summary 85
	4.9	References 85
Chapter 5	Omega-3 Fatty Acids and NO from Flax Intervention in Atherosclerosis and Chronic Systemic Inflammation 89	
	5.1	Atherosclerosis 89
		5.1.1 The Causal Role of ROS in Atherosclerosis 92
		5.1.2 Omega-3 Fatty Acids, an Antioxidant Flaxseed Constituent Can Prevent, Even Reverse, Atherosclerosis 93
		5.1.3 Omega-3 Fatty Acids from Flaxseed 93
		5.1.4 Omega-3 Fatty Acids from Flaxseed and Elevated Blood Cholesterol 94
		5.1.5 Omega-3 Fatty Acids from Flaxseed Lower Triglycerides 96
		5.1.6 L-Arginine (Abundant in Flaxseed) Prevents, Even Reverses, Atherosclerosis 97
	5.2	Chronic Systemic Inflammation 99
		5.2.1 C-Reactive Protein in Inflammation 99
		5.2.2 Omega-3 ALA Reduces Inflammation 101
		5.2.3 L-Arginine, *per se*, and Inflammation 102
		5.2.4 Flax/Omega-3 and Rheumatoid Arthritis 102
	5.3	Summary 103
	5.4	References 104

Chapter 6 Flaxseed and L-Arginine, and Omega-3 Fatty Acids, *per se*, in
Treatment of Hypertension and Sickle Cell Disease 109

6.1 Hypertension 109
    6.1.1 Hypertension as Omega-3 Deficiency 110
    6.1.2 Flax/Omega-3 Fatty Acids Reduces Blood
        Pressure—The Harris Omega-3 Index 111
    6.1.3 The Safety of Cyanogenic Glycosides
        in Flaxseed 113
    6.1.4 L-Arginine Supplementation Reduces Blood
        Pressure 114
    6.1.5 Studies Citing Flaxseed or Flax Oil, *per se*,
        and Hypertension 117
    6.1.6 Could It Be Due to Asymmetric
        Dimethylarginine (ADMA) When
        L-Arginine Fails? 117
        6.1.6.1 Does ADMA Explain the Arginine
                Paradox? 118
6.2 Endothelial Dysfunction in Sickle Cell Disease
    and L-Arginine Therapy 119
6.3 Summary 120
6.4 References 120

Chapter 7 L-Arginine and Omega-3 Fatty Acids in Adjuvant Treatment
for Type 2 Diabetes and Chronic Kidney Disease 125

7.1 The Contribution of Flaxseed Constituents in Type 2
    Diabetes Mellitus 125
    7.1.1 Oxidative Stress in Type 2 Diabetes 126
    7.1.2 Endothelial Dysfunction in Type 2 Diabetes 128
7.2 Flaxseed as Adjuvant Treatment of Type 2 Diabetes 129
    7.2.1 Omega-3 Fatty Acids Reduce Triglycerides in
        Type 2 Diabetes 131
    7.2.2 Type 2 Diabetes and Coronary Heart Disease 132
    7.2.3 Omega-3 Fatty Acid as Adjuvant Treatment of
        Type 2 Diabetes and Nonalcoholic Fatty Liver
        Disease (NAFLD) 132
    7.2.4 Omega-3 Fatty Acid as Adjuvant Treatment of
        Type 2 Diabetes with Diabetic Nephropathy 133
    7.2.5 Treatment Dosage Matters 134
    7.2.6 L-Arginine as Adjuvant Treatment of Type 2
        Diabetes—Is Type 2 Diabetes Mellitus an NO
        Deficiency Disease? 134
7.3 Flax, Inflammation and Endothelium Dysfunction
    in CKD 138
    7.3.1 Flaxseed as Adjuvant Treatment of CKD 138

Contents

		7.3.2	Omega-3 Fatty Acids in Adjuvant Treatment of Kidney Disease...............139
		7.3.3	L-Arginine in Treatment of CKD..............142
		7.3.4	CKD, Hypertension and Chronic Heart Failure........144
	7.4	Summary 145	
	7.5	References...........146	

Chapter 8 NO from Flaxseed Enhances Sexual Function 151

    8.1 Prologue...........151
    8.2 The Oyster and the Blue Pill: Sexual *Desire* vs. Sexual *Performance* 151
        8.2.1 What We Learn from *The Perfumed Garden of the Shaykh Nefzawi* 152
    8.3 The Most Common Cause of Erectile Dysfunction 153
    8.4 Gas Fuels Performance............154
        8.4.1 How a Simple "Blunder" Explains Cardiovascular and Heart Disease 155
    8.5 The Culprit: Oxidative Stress............155
    8.6 The Endothelium Forms Nitric Oxide (eNO)............156
        8.6.1 The Glycocalyx: Sugar Coating the Endothelium 157
    8.7 Sexual Performance Is about *Shunting* Blood Flow in the Body 157
        8.7.1 The Penis Is Not a Muscle 158
    8.8 The (Ach/NO/cGMP) Pathway to Penile Erection 159
    8.9 The Role of Aging in ED............159
        8.9.1 Do We Just Run Out of Gas as We Age?............161
    8.10 Endothelium Dysfunction Is a Feature of ED 162
    8.11 Enter Flaxseed 162
        8.11.1 Flaxseed Supplies L-Arginine, the Substrate for NO 163
        8.11.2 ROS Jeopardize Erectile Function 163
        8.11.3 Flaxseed Supplies the Antioxidant Omega-3 Fatty Acids Promoting eNO Formation 164
    8.12 Summary 166
    8.13 References...........166

Chapter 9 Omega-3 PUFA and L-Arginine for Longer Life Span with a Longer Health Span 169

    9.1 One Way to Longer Life Is to Prevent Shortening It..............169
    9.2 How Can We Tell Whether People Who Consume Flaxseed or Flax Oil Age More Slowly, Live Longer?...........171
        9.2.1 Omega-3s Concentration Affects Cell Aging via Telomere Length...........171

		9.2.2	Omega-3 PUFAs Slow Aging by Lowering Mitochondria Free Radical "Emissions"...................172
		9.2.3	Speaking of Cognitive Aging..174
	9.3	Criteria for Omega-3 Sufficiency: The Omega-3 Index 175	
		9.3.1	Availability vs. Absorbability....................................178
	9.4	Anti-Aging Action of L-Arginine 178	
	9.5	Summary 179	
	9.6	References..180	

Index..183

Preface

In researching publications describing clinical trials or experimental (animal) studies of the effects of flaxseed on medical conditions, we found that the titles of these studies often did not specifically come up with the key word "flaxseed." Given that L-arginine, omega-3 fatty acids and cyanogenic glycosides are three of the main beneficial constituents of flaxseed, we chose to search the literature using those three key words, in addition to the word "flaxseed," in order to detail the medicinal benefits of this plant.

An evidence-based book like this is basically an extended research and clinical studies review. To make it more readable without losing valuable information,

- we omitted the number of participants in treatment or controls groups in any given study unless that information was absolutely vital to understanding the study outcome, e.g., they were either very small or very large in number;
- we substituted the word "significant" for significance levels, usually in the form ($P < 0.05$, or $P < 0.01$);
- we usually left out the type or form of data analysis and the study design, such as double-blind or prospective, unless it was of a special, uncommon type;
- we substituted "participants" or "volunteers" for "subjects";
- we numbered the references instead of citing author/date in the text, e.g., (1), as opposed to (Fried & Carlton, 2018); and
- in some cases, we reproduced (with permission) a large excerpt from given references in order to deepen the reader's grasp of seminal findings that are of particularly key importance.

In addition, in the reference section,

- we list all the authors of a given study,
- we provide the full title of every journal publication, and
- wherever possible, we cited either a DOI or other identifier for ready access to a reference.

Acknowledgments

We express our deep appreciation to Ms. Randy Brehm, Senior Editor, Life Sciences and Nutrition, CRC Press/Taylor & Francis, for, once again, supporting our work, and to Dr. Jacqueline Perle for efficiently carrying out the unenviable task of sorting out and acquiring "permissions."

Disclaimer

The information in this book is neither intended to diagnose nor treat any disease, nor is it a substitute for medical guidance. The authors do not propose that anyone who is undergoing treatment for any medical condition under the care of a physician, or any other qualified healthcare provider, should terminate such treatment in favor of any treatment or substance described here.

Rather, where it may seem helpful to adopt a nutrition strategy based on foods or supplements described here, the authors urge the reader to do so only with the advice, and the supervision, of his or her physician or other qualified healthcare provider.

The information provided here is intended only to educate the reader to what may be available and not to suggest self-treatment. The authors shall not be held liable or responsible for any misunderstanding or misuse of the information contained in this book or for any loss, damage, or injury caused or alleged to be caused directly or indirectly by any treatment, action, or application of any food or food source discussed in this book.

In writing a book that extols the virtues of consuming any given food product for health purposes, there is the risk that others might wonder if the authors gain any commercial benefit from sales of that food or any derivatives thereof. It is therefore important for the reader to know that neither Dr. Fried nor Dr. Carlton, nor any of their relatives or associates, stands to gain financially from sales of flaxseed or any of its derivatives. We are health professionals who have, for scores of years, been seeking out pioneering information in the field of health and nutrition, and have "translated" that pioneering information into books, articles and lectures to make it more accessible and understandable.

1 Introduction

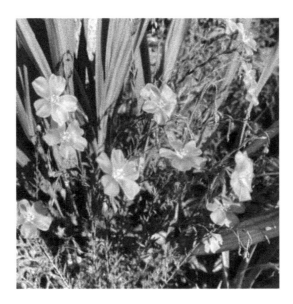

FIGURE 1.1 Flax flowers. (From Nancea Whitham. https://jarvieflora.com/pages/contact-us. With permission.)

All that man needs for health and healing has been provided by God in nature, the challenge of science is to find it.

—**Paracelsus (1493–1541)**

1.1 FLAX—GARMENT OF PHARAOHS AND HEALTH-GIVING SEEDS

Most people driving down a country road probably pay scant attention to the little blue flowers growing by the roadside. These flowers may not have meant much to them at the time. They don't mean much anymore to most people nowadays. In fact, they probably did not even know what the flowers were. Well, they likely were flax flowers, and they actually meant a great deal to our ancestors. Common flax (*Linum usitatissimum* L.) was one of the first domesticated crops. Parenthetically, *usitatissimum* means "most useful." The filaments in their stems were woven into linen (from the Latin word, *linum*); the seeds from their flowers were used as medicine; it was an ingredient in embalming oils.

We use the word "flaxseed" when we consume it as food, whereas we call it "linseed" when it is used in industry or as animal fodder. Flaxseed oil, for instance, is a consumable supplement, whereas linseed oil made from the same flaxseeds is a principal component of commercially produced paint thinners and wood sealers.

There are many claims about the origin and first uses of the flax plant, but it was most likely first cultivated in Mesopotamia possibly as early as 3000 BCE. And through the course of history, the flax plant enjoyed widespread use in ancient Greek cuisine and in ancient Roman medicine, which used it as a laxative, as well as an expectorant for coughs and for soothing irritated tissue.

The linen woven from flax is the world's oldest known textile. The earliest fragment of identified cloth considered to be of linen is from eastern Turkey, carbon-dated to ca. 9,000 years ago. Ancient Egyptian murals and papyri depict the growth of flax, the spinning of flax thread, and the weaving of that thread into linen. And 3,000 to 4,000 years ago, mummified remains of pharaohs were bound in delicate flax linen woven with an expertise that is still difficult to replicate today.

Linen is cited in a number of instances in the Old Testament of the Bible and also in the Gospel of John in connection with the wrappings of the resurrected Lazarus (John 11:1–44). And that use is also illustrated and immortalized in the folk-song lyrics of *Streets of Laredo*, a traditional American Western ballad previously called *A Cowboy's Lament*. Here is the first stanza:

> *As I walked out on the streets of Laredo.*
> *As I walked out on Laredo one day,*
> *I spied a poor cowboy wrapped in white linen,*
> *Wrapped in white linen as cold as the clay.*

In what is now the United States, flax was introduced by the colonists, and it flourished here. But, by the early 20th century, cheaper cotton and rising farm wages had shifted production of flax to northern Russia, which came to provide 90% of the world's output. Since then, flax has lost ground as a commercial crop due to the easy availability of more durable fibers.

Nevertheless, flax still has many uses: it is cultivated for its seeds, which can be ground into meal or turned into flaxseed oil, a nutrition supplement. Flaxseed oil as linseed oil is an ingredient in many wood-finishing products. But flax fibers are still used to make linen, especially fine Belgian flax linen.

To the point, flax holds many constituents, some known as *micronutrients* that are essential to health. It is often suspected that the deficiency of these micronutrients contributes much to the abundance of medical disorders that plague us now, including atherosclerosis, heart failure and chronic kidney disease, type 2 diabetes and many more. These micronutrients are vitamins, minerals and antioxidants needed for healthy living.

Micronutrients are ordinarily contained in common foods we consume, but unfortunately, they are now routinely eliminated in the production of "processed foods" that now constitute much of our food consumption. There is, therefore, a compelling need for supplementation of these micronutrients.

1.2 FLAX—A FUNCTIONAL FOOD

Because of the many health-giving constituents of flax, both in seeds and in oil, it can rightly be considered a "functional food." Functional foods are foods that have

Introduction

a potentially positive effect on health beyond basic nutrition. Proponents of functional foods say they promote optimal health and help reduce the risk of disease. Functional foods differ from *nutraceuticals*. "Nutraceuticals" is a broad umbrella term that is used to describe any products derived from food sources with extra medicinal benefits.

A food that holds one or more nutraceuticals would be considered a functional food. Flax fits that to a "*t*."

This book emphasizes constituents in flax currently considered to be nutraceuticals. The compounds are mainly L-arginine, omega-3 polyunsaturated fatty acids (PUFAs), and cyanogenic glycosides (CNglcs), of which there are three: linamarin, linustatin and neolinustatin.

1.3 CYANOGENIC GLYCOSIDES (CNglcs)

CNglcs are a group of plant nitrate-derived secondary compounds that can yield cyanide (cyanogenesis) following their breakdown by digestive acids and enzymes. They constitute an essential component of plant defense against predatory microbes, fungi and viruses. We know of at least 2,000 plant species that hold CNglcs. Simply put, CNglcs are a combination of cyanide and sugar present in many edible plants (1) including corn, paddy rice, barley, wheat, rye, sugar cane, mango, cassava, lima beans, bamboo shoots, sorghum, flax; common fruits such as apples; and stone fruits like peaches, plums, cherries and apricots. Other sources of dietary cyanide include vitamin B12.

While "cyanogenic glycoside" is a rather daunting, off-putting, unfriendly term that conjures up concerns for safe consumption, these concerns, as you will see, are largely unwarranted.

1.4 HOW SAFE IS IT TO CONSUME FLAXSEED?

Cyanide is a poison, but even so, its toxicity depends entirely on how much of it is consumed. It certainly is not poison when it is formed from CNglcs in the minute quantities found in certain quite common foods. When CNglcs are simply part of the foods consumed, or in the quantity ordinarily contained in recommended servings of flaxseeds or flaxseed oil as nutrient supplements, it is generally considered quite safe to consume.

In fact, flaxseeds have been termed a "functional food" in a report titled "Flax and Flaxseed Oil: An Ancient Medicine and Modern Functional Food" published in the *Journal of Food Science and Technology* in 2014. (2) Countless, perhaps millions of people consume flaxseeds or flaxseed oil every day . . . and live to tell about it—in fact, to acclaim its health benefits.

Although the CNglcs in flaxseeds are essentially the same compound as found in *amygdalin* typically extracted from apricot kernels or the synthetic form, *laetrile*, alleged in the 1950s to cure cancer (and now banned by the Food and Drug Administration [FDA]), its presence in food does not reach the amounts of it consumed in reported attempted cancer "cures" which, in some cases were reported to result in poisoning. (3) But not so CNglcs from flaxseed.

According to a report published in 2017 in the journal *Archives in Cancer Research*, when amygdalin was orally administered to people, the toxic dose was found to be 4 grams per day, for 15 days. (4)

That is far greater than the amount in a serving of flaxseed. Estimates of the amount of ground flaxseed in a tablespoon vary somewhat from source to source, but 6 to 7 grams is the consensus. (5) A report in the journal *Nutrients* tells us that no increase in plasma cyanide levels above baseline has been observed with the consumption of 15 to 100 grams of flaxseeds, which would be about 2 to 16 tablespoons. (6)

The linustatin and neolinustatin found in flaxseed are thought to be the lowest cyanide producers compared to other cyanogenic glycosides. This is because flaxseed glycosides have a molecular structure that resists any spontaneous decomposition to hydrogen cyanide. Theoretically, 1 to 2 tablespoons of flaxseed will produce only approximately 5 to 10 mg of hydrogen cyanide after ingestion. This is highly unlikely to cause toxicity for three reasons:

a) A 50 to 60 mg dose of cyanide is required to cause acute toxicity
b) The human body can routinely detoxify up to 100 mg/day of cyanide (7, 8)
c) By the way, cyanide is heat labile in cooked foods; cooking destroys it (9)

In one study, people given 50 grams/day of flaxseeds did not show increased urinary levels of thiocyanate, a signature metabolite of cyanide. (7) Based on these data, people would need to consume the unrealistic amount of 1 kg of flaxseeds daily for cyanide toxicity to ever manifest itself. (10)

The recommendation of daily dietary supplementation of 9 grams of flaxseed was reported in the *Journal of Food Science and Technology* in connection with its high content of alpha-linolenic acid (ALA; flaxseeds holds about 23 grams/100 grams of ALA). (2) However, Healthline stipulates that supplementation should be kept below 5 tablespoons per day. (11)

The Flax Council of Canada reports that consumption of moderate amounts of flax (1 to 2 tbsp) daily is not likely to pose a health problem for North Americans who have adequate intakes of protein and iodine. (12) In several clinical studies, volunteers ate muffins containing 50 grams (5 to 6 tbsp) of milled flax daily for up to six weeks without ill effects. However, it should be noted that muffins made with milled flax showed no trace of the CNglcs, confirming that cooking destroyed the enzyme that metabolizes CNglcs. (13)

The Flax Council of Canada also noted that there are other sources of dietary cyanide, including a metabolic by-product, *thiocyanates*, which can be found naturally in milk, beer and green vegetables. Thiocyanate is a breakdown product of the CNglcs and of glucosinolates found in millet and in cruciferous vegetables like cabbage, broccoli, cauliflower, kale, mustard, turnip, radish and horseradish.

Thiocyanate can act as a *goitrogen*, meaning that it blocks the uptake of iodine by the thyroid gland. When the diet is overly rich in goitrogens, the thyroid gland swells to trap as much iodine as possible forming a goiter or lump in the neck. The Council notes, however, that there is no evidence that consuming flaxseed produces symptoms of goiter. In fact, goiter is not a health problem where iodine intake is adequate, and it is rare in North America. Goiter occurs mainly in Asia and Africa, and in 96% of cases, it is due to iodine deficiency or consumption of *cassava* and not to the overconsumption of known plant goitrogens. (12)

The Council also noted that flax contains two compounds, phytic acid and oxalate, that bind calcium, copper, iron, magnesium and zinc to form insoluble complexes in the intestine. This may pose a problem for individuals prone to kidney stones. However, flax contains less than 10 mg of oxalate/kgram and about 0.8% to 1.5% phytic acid by seed weight. The amount of phytic acid in flax is comparable to that found in peanuts and soybeans. (14)

To sum up:

> The acute lethal oral dose of cyanide in humans is reported to be between 0.5 and 3.5 mg/kg body weight. The toxic threshold value for cyanide in blood is considered to be between 0.5 (ca. 20 µmol) and 1.0 mg/L (ca. 40 µmol), the lethal threshold value ranges between 2.5 (ca. 100 µmol) and 3.0 mg/L (ca. 120 µmol). 120 grams of crushed/ground flaxseed can be consumed before a toxic threshold of 40 µmol/L is reached. (15)

A tablespoon of milled flaxseed weighs about 10 grams. Thus, to reach the toxic threshold of 40 µmol/L, one would have to consume about 12 tablespoons of milled flaxseed at a sitting.

Furthermore, the safety and benefits of flaxseed are so well-known that it is recommended for heart health and other health reasons by numerous conventional medicine-based websites:

American Heart Association News. "Know the Flax (and the Chia): A Little Seed May Be What Your Diet Needs" (July 19, 2019):

> "Flaxseeds or chia seeds offer good sources of alpha-linolenic acid (ALA), which are unsaturated fatty acids that convert to omega-3 fatty acids typically found in fish," said Linda Van Horn, a registered dietitian and professor in the department of preventive medicine at Northwestern University in Chicago. "But they also offer a good plant-based supply of plant-based proteins, fiber, minerals and other nutrients."

Specifically, flaxseeds contain lignans, a natural chemical compound that along with fiber, antioxidants and healthy fats can help reduce blood cholesterol and may also help lower blood pressure. Some studies suggest lignans may have the potential to reduce tumor growth in women with breast cancer and may protect against prostate cancer." (16)

Mayo Clinic (by Mayo Clinic Staff): "Overview—Polyunsaturated Fat":

> Flaxseed (*Linum usitatissimum*) and flaxseed oil, which comes from flaxseed, are rich sources of the essential fatty acid alpha-linolenic acid—a heart-healthy omega-3 fatty acid. Flaxseed is high in soluble fiber and in lignans, which contain phytoestrogens. Similar to the hormone estrogen, phytoestrogens might have anti-cancer properties. Flaxseed oil doesn't have these phytoestrogens.

Flaxseed can be used whole or crushed, or in a powder form as meal or flour. Flaxseed oil is available in liquid and capsule forms.

Numerous health experts from leading academic centers have made strong recommendations that people use flaxseed and flaxseed oil to reduce cholesterol and blood sugar and to treat diseases of the heart, kidneys and digestive system. A number of these experts also recommend taking flaxseed to treat inflammatory diseases (such as arthritis). (17)

The American Heart Association (AHA) website:

> Polyunsaturated fats can have a beneficial effect on your heart when eaten in moderation and when used to replace saturated fat and trans fat in your diet.

Which foods are high in polyunsaturated fats? Foods high in polyunsaturated fat include a number of plant-based oils, including the following:

- Soybean oil
- Corn oil
- Sunflower oil
- Flaxseed oil

Other sources include some nuts and seeds, such as walnuts and sunflower seeds; tofu; and soybeans. The American Heart Association also recommends eating tofu and other forms of soybeans, canola, walnut and flaxseed and their oils. These foods contain ALA, another omega-3 fatty acid. (18) And, finally:

The *Cleveland Clinic*. "Flaxseed: Little Seed, Big Benefits. How and Why You Should Be Adding Flax to Your Diet":

> Flaxseed benefits. Why do dietitians love flaxseed? Let us count the ways:
> ... Flaxseed is a good source of high-quality plant protein, comparable to soybeans. Potassium. Potassium is a mineral that's important for cell and muscle function and helps maintain normal blood pressure. But many Americans don't get enough.

Enter flaxseed, which has more potassium than (the famously potassium-rich) bananas. (19)

1.5 DISCLAIMER

Flaxseed, flaxseed oil and their individual constituents (omega-3 *alpha*-linolenic acid, L-arginine and trace amounts of cyanogenic glycosides [CNglcs]), with the exception of CNglcs, *per se*, are commonly *independent variables* in the clinical and experimental (animal-model) studies cited in the following chapters. In many cases, they are cited as adjuvant treatment for conditions ranging from heart failure, to diabetes, to chronic kidney disease.

We will list the dosages that are recommended in these studies. But for obvious professional and ethical reasons, we cite these dosages here for information purposes only. We can make no specific recommendations that anyone supplement either a flax product or one of its constituents described in this book without competent medical or other qualified health provider supervision.

While flaxseed and its constituents are generally considered safe as food, not everyone tolerates certain foods, and anaphylaxis is always a possibility. There are also other cases where generally well-tolerated foods or substances can have an unpredicted paradoxical effect. In addition, flaxseed or its constituents supplemented as adjuvant treatment for a serious medical condition cannot be undertaken without exact knowledge of its safety in that setting. This requires on-site medical expertise. We cannot provide that.

L-Arginine, for instance: A clinical study cited in this book found that supplementing L-arginine in a certain kind of kidney transplant significantly improved the treatment outcome except in the case of severe inflammation when, unexpectedly, it had the opposite effect. Furthermore, each of the benefits of flaxseed or its constituents as adjuvant treatment can also constitute a hazard.

1.5.1 CAVEAT

- Flaxseeds or flaxseed oil may result in lowered blood sugar. This may be of concern for individuals with diabetes controlling their blood glucose levels with prescription meds.
- Consuming flaxseed oil may lower blood pressure. This may be of concern for persons who are concurrently taking antihypertensives and/or diuretics.
- The use of flaxseeds may increase the chances of bleeding. This may be of concern for persons concurrently taking certain medications such as anticoagulants ("blood thinners"), including but not limited to aspirin, Coumadin and Plavix.
- Flaxseed and its constituents can affect hormones. This may be of concern for pregnant or lactating women.
- Some people may be allergic to flaxseed or its constituents.
- There is conflicting information about whether ALA in flaxseeds and flaxseed oil causes prostate cancer to become more aggressive. However, flaxseed oil has the nutrient lignan which has been linked to slowing the growth of prostate cancers.

Because flaxseed or its constituents can interfere with the absorption or function of other medications, therefore consultation with a qualified healthcare provider is essential.

1.6 SUPPLEMENT DOSAGES IN CLINICAL AND RESEARCH TRIALS

The 1998 Nobel Prize in Physiology and Medicine was awarded to three American scientists, Drs. Robert F. Furchgott, Louis J. Ignarro and Ferid Murad, who described a physiological phenomenon that no one could have imagined: blood flow throughout the body and the brain is controlled in part by a gas, nitric oxide (NO). NO is an intrinsic vasodilator, formed in and by the endothelial lining of blood vessels. Triggered by the neurotransmitter acetylcholine (Ach), NO formation depends largely on the action of an enzyme, nitric oxide synthase (NOS) on the amino acid L-arginine. More about that in Chapter 8.

When the endothelium is damaged, as is the case, for instance, in hypertension and in atherosclerosis, NO formation may be inadequate, and systemic as well as regional blood flow may be jeopardized. Impaired endothelium NO formation is now seen as the common denominator in most cardiovascular diseases. Thus, restoring that function is now also seen as the key to maintaining or restoring function and, therefore, health. The focus on flaxseed supplementation, then, is that it supports endothelium viability and NO formation and bioavailability:

> First, flaxseed contains omega-3 polyunsaturated fatty acids (PUFAs) that support endothelial function and promote NO formation. In fact, a study titled "Impact of n-3 [omega-3] fatty acids on endothelial function: results from human interventions studies," appeared in the journal *Current Opinion in Clinical Nutrition and Metabolic Care* in 2011. The investigators concluded that *"In individuals with CVD risk factors including overweight, dyslipidemia and Type 2 diabetes n-3 [omega-3] PUFAs may improve endothelial function."* (20)

One tablespoon of ground flax contains 2 g of omega-3s.

Second, flaxseed contains the amino acid L-arginine from which the endothelium derives NO. There is about 2 g of L-arginine per 100 g of basic flaxseed. That's about 1 tablespoon.

Third, flaxseed also contains (very) small amounts of cyanogenic glycosides that likewise contribute to nitric oxide bioavailability.

In sum, there is strong evidence that the constituents of flaxseed, individually, as well as all together, promote cardiovascular health by supporting endothelium viability and supplying the substrate, L-arginine, for nitric oxide formation.

So, the three main relevant ingredients in flaxseed and flaxseed oil supplementation are the omega-3 fatty acid alpha-linoleic acid (ALA) (which the body can convert to eicosapentaenoic acid [EPA] and docosahexaenoic acid [DHA]), L-arginine and cyanogenic glycosides. In the following section, we list the published dosages recommended for omega-3 and L-arginine reported in clinical trials of sole treatment and/or adjuvant treatment of various cardiovascular disorders. There are no published dosages for the use of cyanogenic glycosides (CNglcs) in adjuvant treatment of any conventional medical condition. However, we know that it is present in flaxseed (but not its oil) and that it is a nitric oxide donor (see Chapter 2).

Here are some of the dosages recommended in published clinical reports:

1.6.1 FLAXSEED

- *"1–2 tablespoons a day is considered a healthy amount."* Mar 31, 2015. "Flaxseed Is Nutritionally Powerful"—Mayo Clinic Health System. (www.mayoclinichealthsystem.org; accessed 11/15/21)
- *"30 grams (3 tablespoons equival.) of roasted flaxseed powder for 3 months"* Saxena and Katare. 2014. *Biomedical Journal*, Nov–Dec; 37(6): 386–390. DOI:10.4103/2319–4170.126447.
- *"The amount of flaxseed ingested daily over an extended period of time has been as much as 40 to 50 grams."* Dodin, Lemay, Jacques et al. 2005. *Journal of Clinical Endocrinology and Metabolism*, Mar; 90(3): 1390–1397. DOI:10.1210/ jc.2004–1148.

- "*Human studies with 50 g/day flaxseed did not increase urinary thiocyanate levels.*" Parikh, Netticadan, and Pierce. 2018. *American Journal of Physiology. Heart and Circulatory Physiology*, Feb 1; 314(2): H146-H159. DOI:10.1152/ ajpheart.00400.2017.
- "*Clinical benefits of the n-3 fatty acids were not apparent until they were consumed for > or =12 wk. It appears that a minimum daily dose of 3 g eicosapentaenoic and docosahexaenoic acids is necessary to derive the expected benefits.*" Kremer. 2000. *American Journal of Clinical Nutrition*, Jan; 71(1 Suppl): 349S3–51S. DOI : 10.1093/ajcn/71.1.349s.
- "*Only 10 g of flaxseed in the daily diet increases the daily fiber intake by 1 g of soluble fiber and by 3 g of insoluble fi*ber." Goyal, Sharma, Upadhyay et al. 2014. *Journal of Food Science and Technology*, Sep; 51(9): 1633–1653. DOI:10.1007/ s13197-013-1247-9.
- "*Flaxseed supplementation (30 g/day) on hormonal levels in a 31-year old woman.*" Nowak, Snyder, and Brown. 2007. *Current Topics in Nutraceutical Research*, 5(4): 177–181. PMCID: PMC2752973.

The previous listings are intended to illustrate the range of dosages that clinical investigators consider safe and potentially beneficial in a sample of differing applications.

There is no published recommended dietary allowance for flaxseed or flaxseed oil. But, according to A. Wergin on the Mayo Clinic website, "While there are no specific recommendations for flaxseed intake, 1–2 tablespoons a day is considered a healthy amount." (21) Here are examples of flaxseed dosages in specific clinical applications:

- In treatment of inflammatory biomarkers in patients with coronary artery disease (read endothelial dysfunction): "*12 weeks consumption of flaxseed (30 g/day) or usual care control.*" Khandouzi, Zahedmehr, Mohammadzadeh et al. 2019. Effect of flaxseed consumption on flow-mediated dilation and inflammatory biomarkers in patients with coronary artery disease: a randomized controlled trial. *European Journal of Clinical Nutrition*, Feb; 73(2): 258–265. DOI:10.1038/s41430–018–0268-x.
- In treatment of inflammation in Metabolic Syndrome (read endothelial dysfunction): "*One group received 25 mL/day flaxseed oil.*" Akrami, Makiabadi, Askarpour et al. 2020. A comparative study of the effect of flaxseed oil and sunflower oil on the coagulation score selected oxidative and inflammatory parameters in Metabolic Syndrome patients. *Clinical Nutrition Research*, Jan; 9(1): 63–72. DOI:10.7762/cnr.2020.9.1.63.
- In treatment of dyslipidemia and hypertension: "*The intervention group received 36 g of flaxseed sachet.*" Haghighatsiar, Askari, Saraf-Bank et al. 2019. Effect of flaxseed powder on cardiovascular risk factor in dyslipidemic and hypertensive patients. *International Journal of Preventive Medicine*, 10: 218. DOI:10.4103 /ijpvm.IJPVM_563_17.
- In treatment of dyslipidemia: "*Flaxseed in whole, ground, or defatted form (generically called whole flaxseed) was tested in 10 of 28 trials with doses from 20.0 to 50.0 g (median: 38.0 g; 10 g ≈ 1 tablespoon).*" Pan, Yu,

Demark-Wahnefried et al. 2009. Meta-analysis of the effects of flaxseed interventions on blood lipids. *American Journal of Clinical Nutrition*, Aug; 90(2): 288–297. DOI:10.3945/ajcn.2009.27469.
- In treatment of Type 2 diabetes: "*Type 2 diabetic patients with mild hypercholesterolemia were enrolled into the study. Patients were randomized to supplementation with flaxseed-derived lignan capsules (360 mg lignan per day) or placebo for 12 weeks, separated by an 8-week wash-out period.*" Pan, Sun, Chen et al. 2007. Effects of a flaxseed-derived lignan supplement in type 2 diabetic patients: a randomized, double-blind, crossover trial. *PLoS One*, Nov 7; 2(11): e1148. DOI:10.1371/journal.pone. 0001148.
- In treatment of metabolic syndrome: "*A total of 100 subjects (>or=50 years) were randomized to receive flaxseed lignan (543 mg.day-1 in a 4050 mg complex) or placebo while completing a 6 month walking program (30–60 min.day-1, 5–6 days.week-1).*" Cornish, Chilibeck, Paus-Jennsen et al. 2009. A randomized controlled trial of the effects of flaxseed lignan complex on metabolic syndrome composite score and bone mineral in older adults. *Applied Physiology, Nutrition and Metabolism*, Apr; 34(2): 89–98. DOI:10.1139/H08-142.
- In treatment of blood pressure: "*Hypertriglyceridemic subjects with untreated normal-high blood pressure were prescribed a 2 grams PUFA supplementation.*" Cicero, Derosa, Di Gregori et al. 2010. Omega 3 polyunsaturated fatty acids supplementation and blood pressure levels in hypertriglyceridemic patients with untreated normal-high blood pressure and with or without metabolic syndrome: A retrospective study. *Clinical and Experimental Hypertension*, Jan; 32(2): 137–144. DOI:10.3109/106419609 03254448.
- In prevention of cardiovascular risk factors. "*Men and post-menopausal women with pre-study low density lipoprotein cholesterol (LDL-C) between 130 and 200 mg/dL were randomized to 40 g/day of ground flaxseed-containing baked products or matching wheat bran products for 10 weeks while following a low fat, low cholesterol diet.*" Bloedon, Balikai, Chittams et al. 2008. Flaxseed and cardiovascular risk factors: Results from a double-blind, randomized, controlled clinical trial. *Journal of the American College of Nutrition*, Feb; 27(1): 65–74. DOI:10.1080/07315724.2008. 10719676.
- In treatment of obesity and insulin resistance: "*Nine obese glucose intolerant people consumed 40 g ground flaxseed or 40 g wheat bran daily for 12 weeks with a 4-week washout period.*" Rhee and Brunt. 2011. Flaxseed supplementation improved insulin resistance in obese glucose intolerant people: A randomized crossover design. *Nutrition Journal*, 10: 44. DOI:10.1186/1475-2891-10-44.

According to V. Tan on the Healthline website, "Health benefits . . . were observed with just 1 tablespoon (10 grams) of ground flaxseeds per day. However, it's recommended to keep serving sizes to less than 5 tablespoons (50 grams) of flax seeds per day." (22)

Introduction

CAVEATS
Flaxseed can

- Cause allergy and worsen inflammation
- Be unsafe during pregnancy or lactation
- Cause loose bowels or intestinal blockage
- Interact with medications including those for managing high blood pressure, for thinning the blood and for maintaining healthy blood sugar levels

1.6.2 Omega-3 PUFAs—Alpha-Linolenic Acid (ALA), Eicosapentaenoic Acid (EPA) and Docosahexaenoic Acid (DHA)

Table 1.1 provides information about our understanding of adequate intake of omega-3 fatty acids according to the National Institutes of Health (NIH), Office of Dietary Supplements.

Here is a sample of published clinical and research dosage recommendations:

- *"Current dietary recommendations for adults suggest a daily intake of 2.22 g of ALA based on a 2000 kcal diet."* Rodriguez-Leyva, Bassett, McCullough et al. 2010. *Canadian Journal of Cardiology*, Nov; 26(9): 489–496. DOI:10. 1016/s0828–282x(10)70455–4.
- *"For adults between 25 and 49 years old, Health Canada suggests 1500 mg of omega-3 and 9000 mg of omega-6 polyunsaturates daily for men and 1100 mg of omega-3 and 7000 mg of omega-6 fatty acids daily for women. This results in an omega-6—to—omega-3 ratio of 6:1."* Schwalfenberg. 2006. *Canadian Family Physician*, Jun 10; 52(6): 734–740. PMCID: PMC1780156.

TABLE 1.1
Adequate intake of omega-3 fatty acids

	Adequate Intakes (AIs) for Omega-3s			
Age	Male	Female	Pregnancy	Lactation
Birth to 6 months*	0.5 g	0.5 g		
7–12 months*	0.5 g	0.5 g		
1–3 years**	0.7 g	0.7 g		
4–8 years**	0.9 g	0.9 g		
9–13 years**	1.2 g	1.0 g		
14–18 years**	1.6 g	1.1 g	1.4 g	1.3 g
19–50 years**	1.6 g	1.1 g	1.4 g	1.3 g
51+ years**	1.6 g	1.1 g		

Source: NIH, Office of Dietary Supplements. https://ods.od.nih.gov/factsheets/Omega3 FattyAcids-Health Professional/#h2; accessed 12/1/21.
*As total omega-3s.
**As ALA.

- *"The effects of eicosapentaenoic acid (EPA) 600 and 1800 mg/day and docosahexaenoic acid (DHA) 600 mg/day versus olive oil placebo."* Schaefer, Asztalos, Gleason et al. 2016. *Metabolism*, Nov; 65(11): 1636–1645. DOI:10.1016/j.metabol.2016.07.010.
- *"An Adequate Intake for alpha-linolenic acid, based on the average daily intake by apparently healthy people . . . has been set at 1.6 g/day for adult men and 1.1 g/day for adult women."* Erdman, Oria, and Pillsbury (eds.) 2011. *Nutrition and traumatic brain injury. Improving acute and subacute health outcomes in military personnel.* Chapter 13. Eicosapentaenoic Acid (EPA) and Docosahexaenoic Acid (DHA). Washington DC: National Academies Press. ISBN-13: 978-0-309-21008-9;ISBN-10: 0-309-21008-9. www.ncbi.nlm.nih.gov/books/NBK209320/
- *"In a review of marketed fish oil supplements (110 non-liquid and 14 liquid), the median amount of EPA/DHA in non-liquid and liquid products was 0.216 g/0.2 g and 0.46 g/0.4 g, respectively.* Therefore, in order to achieve a dose of 3.36 g/day omega-3 fatty acids, it was found that a median intake of 11.2 servings/day would be required at a median monthly cost of $63.49 for non-liquid formulations, and a median 3.6 teaspoons/day would be required at a median monthly cost of $13.60 for liquid formulations."* Bradberry, and Hilleman. 2013. *Pharmacy and Therapeutics*, Nov; 38(11): 681–691. PMCID: PMC3875260.

The preceding listing is intended to illustrate the range of dosages that are considered safe and potentially effective in a sample of differing clinical applications.

Table 1.2 lists ALA, EPA and DHA content of selected foods according to the US Department of Agriculture, Agricultural Research Service, FoodData Central, 2019.

Here are some examples of omega-3 PUFA dosage in specific applications:

- Example of omega-3 dosage in treatment of endothelial dysfunction: *"Healthy volunteers . . . were given supplementation at 4g/day omega-3 fatty acids (or were not treated) for 4 weeks."* Miyoshi, Noda, and Ohno. 2014. Omega-3 fatty acids improve postprandial lipemia and associated endothelial dysfunction in healthy individuals—a randomized crossover trial. *BioMed Pharmacotherapy*, Oct; 68(8): 1071–1077. DOI:10.1016/j.biopha.2014.10.008.
- Example of omega-3 dosage in treatment of heart disease: *"Patients surviving recent (< or = 3 months) myocardial infarction were randomly assigned supplements of n-3 PUFA 1 g daily . . ."* No authors listed. 1999. Dietary supplementation with n-3 polyunsaturated fatty acids and vitamin E after myocardial infarction: Results of the GISSI-Prevenzione Trial. Gruppo Italiano per lo Studio della Sopravvivenza nell'Infarto miocardico. *Lancet*, Aug 7; 354(9177):4 47–455. PMID: 10465168.
- Example of omega-3 dosage in treatment of coronary heart disease: *"In patients with coronary heart disease the guidelines recommend 1 g daily supplements and in hypertriglyceridaemic patients up to 4 g per day."* Mori. 2014. Omega-3 fatty acids and cardiovascular disease: Epidemiology and effects on cardiometabolic risk factors. *Food and Function*, Sep; 5(9): 2004–2019. DOI:10.1039/c4fo 00393d.

---

* It is not obvious to us what the authors mean by "0.216 g/0.2 g and 0.46 g/0.4 g." We are quoting them directly.

TABLE 1.2
ALA, EPA and DHA content of selected foods

Food	Grams per Serving		
	ALA	DHA	EPA
Flaxseed oil, 1 tbsp	7.26		
Chia seeds, 1 ounce	5.06		
English walnuts, 1 ounce	2.57		
Flaxseed, whole, 1 tbsp	2.35		
Salmon, Atlantic, farmed cooked, 3 ounces		1.24	0.59
Salmon, Atlantic, wild, cooked, 3 ounces		1.22	0.35
Herring, Atlantic, cooked, 3 ounces*		0.94	0.77
Canola oil, 1 tbsp	1.28		
Sardines, canned in tomato sauce, drained, 3 ounces*		0.74	0.45
Mackerel, Atlantic, cooked, 3 ounces*		0.59	0.43
Salmon, pink, canned, drained, 3 ounces*	0.04	0.63	0.28
Soybean oil, 1 tbsp	0.92		
Trout, rainbow, wild, cooked, 3 ounces		0.44	0.40
Black walnuts, 1 ounce	0.76		
Mayonnaise, 1 tbsp	0.74		
Oysters, eastern, wild, cooked, 3 ounces	0.14	0.23	0.30
Sea bass, cooked, 3 ounces*		0.47	0.18
Edamame, frozen, prepared, ½ cup	0.28		
Shrimp, cooked, 3 ounces*		0.12	0.12
Refried beans, canned, vegetarian, ½ cup	0.21		
Lobster, cooked, 3 ounces*	0.04	0.07	0.10
Tuna, light, canned in water, drained, 3 ounces*		0.17	0.02
Tilapia, cooked, 3 ounces*	0.04	0.11	
Scallops, cooked, 3 ounces*		0.09	0.06
Cod, Pacific, cooked, 3 ounces*		0.10	0.04
Tuna, yellowfin, cooked 3 ounces*		0.09	0.01
Kidney beans, canned ½ cup	0.10		
Baked beans, canned, vegetarian, ½ cup	0.07		
Ground beef, 85% lean, cooked, 3 ounces**	0.04		
Bread, whole wheat, 1 slice	0.04		
Egg, cooked, 1 egg		0.03	
Chicken, breast, roasted, 3 ounces		0.02	0.01
Milk, low-fat (1%), 1 cup	0.01		

Source: US Department of Agriculture (USDA), Agricultural Research Service. FoodData Central, 2019.
*Except as noted, the USDA database does not specify whether fish are farmed or wild caught.
**The USDA database does not specify whether beef is grass fed or grain fed.

- Example of omega-3 dosage in treatment of type 2 diabetes: *"Group II received metformin 500 mg twice daily and omega-3 fatty acids (1 gram) once daily."* Chauhan, Kodali, Noor et al. 2017. Role of omega-3 fatty acids on lipid profile in diabetic dyslipidaemia: Single blind, randomized clinical trial. *Journal of*

Clinical and Diagnostic Research, Mar; 11(3): OC13—OC16. DOI:10.7860/JCDR/2017/20628.9449.
- Example of omega-3 dosage in treatment of kidney function and myocardial infarction: "*The patients received an additional targeted amount of 400 mg/d eicosapentaenoic acid and docosahexaenoic acid, 2 g/d α-linolenic acid, eicosapentaenoic acid—docosahexaenoic acid plus α-linolenic acid.*" Hoogeveen, and Geleijnse. 2014. Effect of omega-3 fatty acids on kidney function after myocardial infarction: The Alpha Omega trial. *Clinical Journal of the American Society of Nephrology*, Oct 7; 9(10): 1676–1683. DOI:10.2215/CJN.10441013.
- Example of omega-3 dosage in treatment of inflammation in chronic kidney disease (CKD): "*Six-month supplementation with omega-3 acids (2 g/day) was administered to 87 CKD patients.*" Pluta, Stróżecki, and Kęsy. 2017. Beneficial effects of 6-month supplementation with omega-3 acids on selected inflammatory markers in patients with chronic kidney disease stages 1–3. *BioMed Research International*, 2017: 1680985. Published online 2017 Nov 19. DOI:10.1155/2017/1680985.
- In treatment of metabolic syndrome: "*Were administered 1.7 g of [Long-chain omega-3 fatty acids from fish oils] O3 per day . . . or safflower oil placebo.*" Root, Collier, Zwetsloot et al. 2013. A randomized trial of fish oil omega-3 fatty acids on arterial health, inflammation, and metabolic syndrome in a young healthy population. *Nutrition Journal*, 2013 Apr 8; 12: 40. DOI:10.1186/1475-2891-12-40. There are, in addition, FDA-approved omega-3 PUFAs supplements for adults 18 years old or older with hypertriglyceridemia ($\geq$ 500 mg/dL) as an adjunct to diet and exercise.
- Icosapent ethyl is administered as capsules with a daily dose of 4 g/day taken as two, 2-gram capsules twice a day with meals.
- Omega-3-acid ethyl esters are administered as capsules with a daily dose of 4 g/day taken as four capsules once a day with meals or two capsules twice a day with meals.
- *Omega-3-carboxylic acids* are administered as capsules with a daily dose of 2 g/day taken as two capsules once per day or 4 g/day taken as four capsules once a day. Clinical trial administration was without regard to meals.
- Ome*ga-3-acid ethyl esters A* are administered as capsules with a daily dose of 4 g/day taken as four capsules once a day with meals or two capsules twice a day with meals. (23)

Parenthetically, Vascepa and Lovaza are two prescription brand-name omega-3 fatty acid medications that treat high triglyceride levels. Both medicines are approved by the US FDA.

1.6.3 L-Arginine

L-arginine, the substrate for endothelial nitric oxide (eNO) formation, is a conditionally essential amino acid, which means that it is usually not essential except in times of

Introduction

illness and stress. Conditionally essential amino acids include also cysteine, glutamine, tyrosine, glycine, ornithine, proline and serine.

Mean dietary L-arginine intake by US adults is reported to be 4.40 g/day, with 25% of people consuming less than 2.6 g/day. (24) Median L-arginine intake in the adult population, participants of the National Health Nutrition and Examination Survey, was also estimated to be 3.8 g/day. The highest level (90th percentile) of intake of L-arginine in our population (6.7 g/day) was also within the range of previous reports (4.5–7.5 g/day). (25)

Here is a sample of published clinical and research dosage recommendations:

- *"Healthy men received L-arginine supplementation (2000 mg daily) in the intervention group . . . for 45 days."* Pahlavani, Jafari, Sadeghi et al. 2014. *F1000 Research*, 3: 306. DOI:10.12688/f1000research.5877.2.
- *"Patients . . . receive[d] either L-arginine (3 or 6 g thrice daily) or placebo for 8 weeks."* Dashtabi, Mazloom, Fararouei et al. 2015. *Research in Cardiovascular Medicine*, Dec 29; 5(1): e29419. DOI:10.5812/cardiovascmed.29419.
- *"Athletes received daily either 2 g per day l-arginine supplement or the same amount of placebo (maltodextrin) for 45 days."* Pahlavani N, Entezari MH, Nasiri M, Miri A, Rezaie M, Bagheri-Bidakhavidi M, and O Sadeghi. 2017. *European Journal of Clinical Nutrition*, Apr; 71(4):544–548. DOI:10.1038/ejcn.2016.266.
- *"Intravenous infusion of 30 g and 6 g l-arginine."* Bode-Böger, Böger, Galland et al. 1998. *British Journal of Clinical Pharmacology*, Nov; 46(5): 489–497. DOI:10.1046/j.1365–2125.1998.00803.x.
- *"Healthy young men 27 to 37 years old took L-arginine (7 g three times daily) or placebo for 3 days each."* Adams, Forsyth, Jessup et al. 1995. *Journal of the American College of Cardiology*, Oct; 26(4): 1054–1061. DOI:10.1016/0735–1097 (95)00257–9.
- *"Each subject was studied before and after 4 wk of L-arginine (7 grams x 3/day) or placebo powder."* Clarkson, Adams, Powe et al. 1996. *Journal of Clinical Investigation*, Apr 15; 97(8): 1989–1994. DOI:10.1172/JCI118632. DOI:10.1172 /JCI118632.

Here are published examples of L-arginine dosage in specific applications:

- In treatment of endothelial dysfunction: *"L-arginine (8 g p.o. two times daily) or placebo for 14 days each."* Bode-Böger, Muke, Surdacki et al. 2003. Oral L-arginine improves endothelial function in healthy individuals older than 70 years. *Vascular Medicine*, May; 8(2): 77–81. DOI:10.1191/13 58863x03vm474oa.
- In treatment of heart disease: *"Healthy men received L-arginine supplementation (2000 mg daily) in the intervention group."* Pahlavani, Jafari, Sadeghi et al. 2017. L-Arginine supplementation and risk factors of cardiovascular diseases in healthy men: A double-blind randomized clinical trial. F1000Res, 3: 306. DOI:10.12688/f1000research.5877.2.

- As an antioxidant in treatment of patients with angina or following myocardial infarction: *"L-arginine administration (three grams per day for 15 days) resulted in increased activity of free radical scavenging enzyme superoxide dismutase (SOD) and increase in the levels of total thiols (T-SH) and ascorbic acid with concomitant decrease in lipid per-oxidation, carbonyl content, serum cholesterol and the activity of proxidant enzyme, xanthine oxidase (XO)."* Tripathi, Chandra, and Misra. 2009. Oral administration of L-arginine in patients with angina or following myocardial infarction may be protective by increasing plasma superoxide dismutase and total thiols with reduction in serum cholesterol and xanthine oxidase. *Oxidative Medicine and Cell Longevity*, Sep–Oct; 2(4): 231–237. DOI:10.4161/oxim.2.4.9233.
- In treatment of obese, insulin-resistant type 2 diabetic patients: *"The first group was also treated with L-arginine (8.3 g/day)."* Lucotti, Setola, and Monti. 2006. Beneficial effects of a long-term oral L-arginine treatment added to a hypocaloric diet and exercise training program in obese, insulin-resistant type 2 diabetic patients. *American Journal of Physiology, Endocrinology and Metabolism*, Nov; 291(5): E906–12. DOI:10.1152/ajpendo.00002.2006.
- In treatment of chronic renal failure (CRF): *"Patients received either L-arginine (300 mg/kg) or placebo."* Miller, Dascalu, and Rassin. 2003. Effects of an acute dose of L-arginine during coronary angiography in patients with chronic renal failure. A randomized, parallel, double-blind clinical trial. *American Journal of Nep*hrology, 23: 91–95. DOI: https://doi.org/10.1159/000068036.
- In treatment of sickle cell disease with vaso-occlusive pain episodes: *"Patients received L-arginine (100 mg/kg tid) or placebo for 5 days or until discharge."* Morris, Kuypers, and Lavrisha. 2013. A randomized, placebo-controlled trial of arginine therapy for the treatment of children with sickle cell disease hospitalized with vaso-occlusive pain episodes. *Haematologica*, Sep; 98(9): 1375–1382. DOI:10.3324/haematol.2013.086637.
- In treatment of Peripheral Artery Disease (PAD): *"Patients were randomly assigned to oral doses of 0, 3, 6 or 9 g of L-arginine daily in three divided doses for 12 weeks."* Oka, Szuba, and Giacomini. 2005. A pilot study of L-arginine supplementation on functional capacity in peripheral arterial disease. *Vascular Medicine*, Nov; 10(4): 265–274. DOI:10.1191/1358863x05vm637oa.
- In treatment of intermittent claudication: *"Thirty-nine patients with intermittent claudication were randomly assigned to receive 2 x 8 g L-arginine/day."* Böger, Bode-Böger, Thiele et al. 1998. Restoring vascular nitric oxide formation by L-arginine improves the symptoms of intermittent claudication in patients with peripheral arterial occlusive disease. *Journal of the American College of Cardiology*, Nov; 32(5): 1336–1344. DOI:10.1016/s0735-1097(98)00375-1.
- In treatment of erectile dysfunction (ED): *"The analysis demonstrated that arginine supplements with dosage ranging from 1,500 to 5,000 mg significantly improved ED compared with placebo or no treatment."* Rhim,

Kim, Park et al. 2019. The potential role of arginine supplements on erectile dysfunction: A systemic review and meta-analysis. *Journal of Sexual Medicine*, Feb; 16(2): 223–234. DOI:10.1016/j.jsxm. 2018.12.002.

CAVEAT
Possible interactions of L-arginine with medications include the following:

- *Anticoagulants and anti-platelet drugs, herbs and supplements.* Some examples of these types of products (drugs, herbs and supplements) can reduce blood clotting. Taking L-arginine with them might potentiate them, thereby increasing the risk of bleeding.
- *Blood pressure drugs, herbs and supplements.* L-Arginine might lower blood pressure in people who have high blood pressure. Therefore combining L-arginine with a blood pressure-lowering drug, herb or supplement might increase the risk of blood pressure becoming too low.
- *Diabetes drugs, herbs and supplements.* L-Arginine might decrease blood sugar levels in people with diabetes. Taking anti-diabetes drugs, herbs or supplements may require adjusting the dosage of meds.
- *Isoproterenol (Isuprel).* Use of this heart medication with L-arginine might cause low blood pressure.
- *Nitrates.* Use of this chest pain medication with L-arginine might cause low blood pressure. Diuretics (potassium-sparing diuretics). One should not take L-arginine with amiloride (Midamor), spironolactone (Aldactone, Carospir) or triamterene (Dyrenium). These medications can increase potassium levels, raising the risk of developing a higher than normal blood levels of potassium.
- *Sildenafil (Revatio, Viagra) and tadafil.* Use of this erectile dysfunction medication with L-arginine might cause a precipitous fall in blood pressure.

There is no standard dose of arginine. Studies have used different amounts for different conditions. One common dosage is 2 to 3 grams three times a day, although lower and higher doses have also been studied. The safety of long-term L-arginine supplement use is not clear. (26)

Although higher doses are often used in research and clinical settings, it is recommended by some authorities that daily dosing of L-arginine be kept under 9 grams per day to avoid potential gastrointestinal side effects. (27)

In 2018, the journal *Amino Acids* published a report titled "Safety of Dietary Supplementation with Arginine in Adult Humans." The investigators reported that previous studies have shown beneficial effects of dietary supplementation with L-arginine (Arg) on reducing white fat and improving health but that long-term safe levels administered to people are unknown. Therefore, the aim of their study was to evaluate the safety and tolerability of oral L-arginine in overweight or obese but otherwise healthy adults with a body mass index of ≥ 25 kg/m2.

A total of 142 participants completed a 7-day wash-in period using a 12 g Arg/day dose. All the remaining eligible participants who tolerated the wash-in dose were then assigned to 0, 15 or 30 g Arg (as pharmaceutical-grade Arg-HCl) per day for 90 days. The L-arginine treatment was taken daily in at least two divided doses by mixing it with a flavored beverage.

At Days 0 and 90, blood pressures of treatment participants were recorded, their physical examinations were performed and their blood and 24-hour urine samples were obtained to measure the serum concentrations of amino acids, glucose, fatty acids and related metabolites; and the renal, hepatic, endocrine and metabolic parameters.

It was found that the serum concentration of Arg in men or women significantly increased progressively with increasing oral Arg doses from 0 to 30 g/day. Dietary supplementation with 30 g Arg/day significantly reduced systolic blood pressure and serum glucose concentration in women, as well as serum concentrations of free fatty acids in both men and women.

It seems that the treatment participants tolerated oral administration of 15 and 30 g Arg/day without adverse events. And, it is concluded that a long-term safe level of dietary Arg supplementation is at least 30 g/day in adults. (28)

1.7 AD LIB SUPPLEMENTATION

There is a difference between supplementation and adjuvant treatment. It is assumed that the individual who wants to supplement is looking to harvest the health benefits of a given supplement, whereas in adjuvant treatment, there is a medical prescription treatment plan in place. As noted earlier, supplements may interact with prescription meds, possibly with adverse consequences. That said, supplementation of flaxseed and flaxseed oil is popular. Here is a market review report from Grand View Research, San Francisco, CA 94105:

> *The global flaxseeds market size was valued at USD 423.3 million in 2018 and is expected to expand at a CAGR of 12.7% over the forecast period. Growing awareness related to the health benefits of linseed is the main factor anticipated to drive the market over the forecast period.* (29)

Should one buy organic or nonorganic flaxseeds? According to the Flax Council of Canada, all flax that is "clean and that comes from a reputable supplier" is considered to be safe for consumption.

- *Whole flaxseeds*—Flaxseed eaten whole supplies the benefits of the fiber and the lignans. In order to benefit from the omega 3-fatty acid in the flaxseeds, the seeds must be chewed well or ground. Whole flaxseeds can be stored at room temperature for up to 10 months.
- *Ground flaxseeds or flax meal*—There are approximately 1.6 grams of omega 3-fatty acids in 1 tbsp of ground flaxseeds. When it is eaten ground, all nutritional benefits, i.e., omega 3-fatty acids, fiber, and lignans, in flaxseeds are preserved. Ground flaxseeds are best stored in the refrigerator or freezer and for no longer than 3 months. If one grinds the seeds, it is best to grind as needed to prevent spoilage.
- *Flax oil*—Flax oil is extracted from the whole flax seed. It is sold as oil or in gel supplements. It is best to keep flax oil in a cool, dark place—ideally in the refrigerator. Flax oil is an excellent source of omega 3-fatty acids, but it contains neither the lignans nor the fiber, as these are eliminated in the

Introduction

process of oil extraction. One can look at the manufacturer's best-before date to determine how long it can be stored. There are approximately 7.2 grams of omega 3-fatty acids in 1 tbsp of flax oil.

To obtain the benefits of the entire flaxseed, the best way to consume it is in the form of the ground (or milled) flaxseed/flax meal. (30)

1.7.1 RAW FLAXSEED

According to the Healthline website, consuming whole or ground flaxseed delivers all three macronutrients: carbohydrates, protein and fat. When comparing golden flaxseed with brown flaxseed, the exact amount of protein, fat and carbohydrates will depend on the type chosen.

Most adults are likely to consume about an ounce (28 grams) of whole or ground flaxseeds per serving and, according to the US Department of Agriculture (USDA), this amount of flaxseed contains the following:

- 152 calories
- 12 grams of fat
- 8.2 grams of carbohydrates, 7.8 grams of which come from dietary fiber
- 5.2 grams of protein
- 6% of the daily value (DV) for calcium
- 9% of the DV for iron
- 5% of the DV for potassium
- 27% of the DV for magnesium
- 15% of the DV for phosphorus
- 11% of the DV for zinc
- 38% of the DV for copper
- 31% of the DV manganese
- 13% of the DV for selenium
- 39% of the DV for thiamin (vitamin B1)
- 5 % of the DV for niacin (vitamin B3)
- 6% of the DV for vitamin B5
- 8% of the DV for vitamin B6
- 6% of the DV for folic acid (vitamin B9)

Flaxseeds are also rich in lutein and zeaxanthin, antioxidants like phenolic compounds and flavonoids and lignans, a type of polyphenol. You can also find small amounts (between 1% and 4%) of B-complex vitamins, vitamin E, vitamin K and choline in each ounce of flaxseeds.

Parenthetically, most of these nutrients are not present in flaxseed oil. Flaxseed oil and capsules contain pure fat and lack most of the nutritional value that whole and ground flaxseed products contain. (31)

Golden flaxseed vs. brown flaxseed—the difference between golden and brown flaxseed is minimal and centers on their macronutrient and antioxidant contents. Golden flaxseed is made up of about 37.5% fat, 23% protein and 30%

carbohydrates, while brown flaxseed is made up of 38% fat, 24.5% protein and 28% carbohydrates. However, what is different between golden and brown flaxseed is the type of fat in each.

Golden flaxseeds have more polyunsaturated fatty acids and less monounsaturated fatty acids compared to brown flaxseeds. They also have larger amounts of the two *essential* fats, i.e., *alpha*-linolenic acid (ALA) and linoleic acid present in different ratios in golden and brown flaxseed. There is more ALA in golden flaxseed than linoleic acid.

Most people who follow a Western Diet typically consume too many omega-6 fats, like linoleic acid, and not enough omega-3 fats, like ALA. For that reason, golden flaxseed is a better choice for supplementing the diet with healthy fats. However, brown flaxseed has a substantially higher concentration of antioxidants. In fact, compared to other similar seeds, like chia seeds and perilla seeds, golden flaxseeds are always the lowest in antioxidants. (32) Perilla, by the way, is a kind of mint.

Flaxseed can readily be purchased in health food stores and online. For example[*]:

- Bob's Red Mill Organic Flax Seed
- Spectrum Essentials Organic Ground Premium
- Premium Gold Whole Flax Seed
- FGO Whole Brown Flaxseed
- Anthony's Organic Flaxseed Meal

What type of flaxseed is healthiest? Most nutrition experts recommend ground over whole flaxseed because the ground form is easier to digest. Whole flaxseed may pass through your intestine undigested, which means you won't get all the benefits.

Examples of ground flaxseed:

- Premium Gold Organic Ground Flax Seed
- Spectrum Essentials Organic Ground Flaxseed
- Viva Naturals Organic Ground Flax Seed
- Anthony's Organic Flaxseed Meal
- Terrasoul Superfoods Organic Ground Flax Seeds

Whole seeds can be ground at home using a coffee grinder or food processor. For instance:

- COOL KNIGHT Herb Grinder Electric Spice Grinder (electric)
- Cuisinart SG-10 Electric Spice-and-Nut Grinder (electric)
- Mini Seed Mill & Coffee Grinder (electric)
- Glass Sesame Seed Grinder by Asvel (hand power)
- Staub Cast Iron Grinder (hand power)

---

[*] We have no financial interest in any commercial product(s) cited in this book, which are offered simply as an example of what is available. Nor does any citation constitute an endorsement. We cannot certify any representation by a product manufacturer as to quality, purity or efficacy of the product(s).

1.7.2 Including Flaxseed in Daily Diet

- Add a tablespoon of ground flaxseed to hot or cold breakfast cereal.
- Add a teaspoon of ground flaxseed to mayonnaise or mustard when making a sandwich.
- Mix a tablespoon of ground flaxseed into an 8-ounce container of yogurt.
- Bake ground flaxseed into cookies, muffins, breads and other baked goods.

Like other sources of fiber, flaxseed should be taken with plenty of water or other fluids. Flaxseed shouldn't be taken at the same time as oral medications. (33)

One can also find a number of recipes online for including flaxseed in meals. For instance: Flaxseed recipes—these flaxseed-based recipes are a great place to help weight loss and health goals. Start with one recipe each day to reap the benefits.

Adding flaxseed to oatmeal, smoothies and yogurt bowls is a great way to add protein, fiber and texture to your dish. Get started with one of these easy recipes.

- Flaxseed and blueberry oatmeal
- High-protein strawberry flax smoothie
- Chia and flax seed breakfast bowl
- Apple pie overnight oats
- Low-carb yogurt parfait with strawberries, flax and chia seeds

Flaxseed breads, tortillas, muffins and loaf recipes:

- Chia and flaxseed tortillas
- Flax, carrot, apple muffins
- Healthy oatmeal chocolate chip cookies
- Flaxseed meal pancakes
- Honey flax banana bread

Flaxseed snack recipes:

- No-bake energy bites
- Honey almond flax granola
- Easy crunch flaxseed crackers
- Flaxseed apricot bars
- Power biscotti

Other flaxseed recipes:

- Healthy baked turkey meatballs
- Flaxseed chicken tenders
- Almond flax crusted fish
- Veggie-flax burgers
- Keto low-carb meatballs*

---

* Source: 25 Simple Flaxseed Recipes by noom | Sep 20, 2019.

- TopTeenRecipes—16 Easy Flaxseed Recipes: https://topteenrecipes.com/flaxseed-recipes/
- EatingWell—Healthy Flax Seed Recipes: www.eatingwell.com/recipes/19239/ingredients/nuts-seeds/flax-seed/
- CookingLight—15 Ways to Use Ground Flaxseed: www.cookinglight.com/food/recipe-finder/ground-flaxseed-recipes
- Profusion Curry—Flaxseed Garlic Chutney—Superfoods Chutney: https://profusioncurry.com/flaxseed-garlic-chutney-superfoods-chutney/
- Flaxseed Bread: https://nutritionrefined.com/flaxseed-bread/

There are also books with flaxseed recipes:

- Michelle Bakema M. 2015. *Flaxseed Recipes: Lose Weight, Gain Energy, & Achieve Overall Wellness.* CreateSpace Independent Publishing Platform.
- Gale Spratley G. 2021. *The Ultimate Guide To Flaxseed: Making Recipes for Breakfast, Smoothie, Soup, Desserts, and More: Ground Flaxseed Recipes.* Independently Published.
- Bloomfield B, Judy Brown J, and S Gursche. 2000. *Flax the Super Food!: Over 80 Delicious Recipes Using Flax Oil and Ground Flaxseed (Over 80 Delicious Recipes Using Flax Oil & Ground Flaxseed).* Kindle Edition. Book Publishing Company (TN).
- Vincent E. 2013. *Flaxseed Recipes: How to Use Flaxseed in Omega 3, Low Carb, Wheat Free, Egg Free, Celiac Disease and Gluten Free Recipes. Includes 36 Flax Seed Recipes.* Kindle Edition. Sidewinder Media.
- Niles S. 2014. *Flaxseed Recipes: 50 Delicious Recipes Using Flaxseed to Reduce Weight and Firing Up Your Metabolism rate.* Paperback. CreateSpace Independent Publishing Platform.

1.8 SUMMARY

There is a long history of mankind's use of flax in many different ways as food, medicine, and in making fine cloth. Flaxseed is a functional food that supplies basic health-giving nutrients: The omega-3 fatty acids it contains are antioxidants that also help to control weight, blood pressure, cholesterol levels and protect the vascular endothelium. It also contains the amino acid L-arginine, the substrate for the formation of endothelial NO, an intrinsic vasodilator that helps regulate blood flow throughout the body. In addition, flaxseed contains very small quantities of CNglcs that also contribute to the formation of NO. There are different varieties of flaxseed that differ from each other in small ways, and there are different ways of consuming flaxseed as a dietary supplement. We cite examples of websites and books that supply recipes.

1.9 REFERENCES

1. Bolarinwa IF, Oke MO, Olaniyan SA, and AS Ajala. 2016. A review of cyanogenic glycosides in edible plants. *Toxicology*. London: IntechOpen, Oct 26. DOI:10.5772/64886.

2. Goyal A, Sharma V, Upadhyay N, Gill S, and M Sihag. 2014. Flax and flaxseed oil: An ancient medicine and modern functional food. *Journal of Food Science and Technology*, Sep; 51(9): 1633–1653. DOI:10.1007/s13197-013-1247-9.
3. Dang T, Nguyen C, and PN Tran. 2017. Physician beware: Severe cyanide toxicity from amygdalin tablets ingestion. *Case Report in Emergency Medicine*, 2017: 4289527. DOI: 10.1155/2017/4289527.
4. Qadir M, and K Fatima. 2017. Review on pharmacological activity of amygdalin. *Archives in Cancer Research*, 5(4): 160. DOI:10.21767/2254-6081.100160.
5. Nutrition and Healthy Eating. www.mayoclinic.org/healthy-lifestyle/nutrition-and-healthy-eating/expert-answers/flaxseed/faq-20058354; accessed 1/7/20.
6. Cressey P, and J Reeve. 2019. Metabolism of cyanogenic glycosides: A review. *Food and Chemical Toxicology*, Mar; 125: 225–232. DOI:10.1016/j.fct.2019.01.002.
7. Parikh M, Netticadan T, and GB Pierce. 2018. Flaxseed: Its bioactive components and their cardiovascular benefits. *American Journal of Physiology. Heart and Circulation Physiology*, Feb; 314(2): H146–H159. DOI:10.1152/ajpheart.00400.2017.
8. Touré A, and X Xueming. 2019. Flaxseed lignans: Source, biosynthesis, metabolism, antioxidant activity, bio-active components, and health benefits. *Comprehensive Reviews in Food Science and Food Safety*, May; 9: 261–269. DOI:10.1111/j.1541-4337.2009.00105.x.
9. Kajla P, Sharma A, and DR Sood. 2015. Flaxseed-a potential functional food source. *Journal of Food Science and Technology*, Apr; 52(4): 1857–1871. DOI:10.1007/s13197-014-1293-y.
10. Parikh M, Maddaford TG, Austria A, Aliani M, Netticadan T, and GN Pierce1. 2019. Dietary flaxseed as a strategy for improving human health. *Nutrients*, May; 11(5): 1171. DOI:10.3390/nu11051171.
11. www.healthline.com/nutrition/benefits-of-flaxseeds; accessed 1/7/20.
12. Morris DH. 2007. *Flax: A health and nutrition primer*, 4th ed., Chapter 8. Safety of Flax. https://flaxcouncil.ca/wp-content/uploads/2015/03/FlxPrmr_4ed_Chpt8.pdf.
13. Cunnane SC, Ganguli S, Menard C, Liede AC, Hamadeh MJ, Chen ZY, Wolever TM, and DJ Jenkins. 1993. High α-linolenic acid flaxseed (*Linum usitatissimum*): Some nutritional properties in humans. *British Journal of Nutrition*, 69: 443–453.
14. Whitney EN, and SR Rolfes. 2005. *Understanding nutrition*, 10th ed. Belmont, CA: Wadsworth.
15. Schrenk D, Bignami M, Bodin L, Kevin Chipman JK, del Mazo J, Grasl-Kraupp B, Hogstrand C, Hoogenboom L(R), Leblanc J-C, Nebbia CS, Nielsen E, Ntzani E, Petersen A, Sand S, Vleminckx C, Wallace H, Benford D, Brimer L, Mancini FR, Metzler M, Viviani B, Altieri A, Arcella D, Steinkellner H, and T Schwerdtle. 2019. Evaluation of the health risks related to the presence of cyanogenic glycosides in foods other than raw apricot kernels EFSA Panel on Contaminants in the Food Chain (CONTAM), *EFSA Journal*, 17(4): 5662. DOI:10.2903/j.efsa.2019.5662.
16. www.heart.org/en/news/2019/07/19/know-the-flax-and-the-chia-a-little-seed-may-be-what-your-diet-needs; accessed 11/15/21.
17. www.mayoclinic.org/drugs-supplements-flaxseed-and-flaxseed-oil/art-20366457; accessed 5/12/21.
18. www.heart.org/en/healthy-living/healthy-eating/eat-smart/fats/polyunsaturated-fats; accessed 11/15/21.
19. https://health.clevelandclinic.org/flaxseed-little-seed-big-benefits/; accessed 11/15/21.
20. Egert S, and P Stehle. 2011. Impact of n-3 fatty acids on endothelial function: Results from human interventions studies. *Current Opinion in Clinical Nutrition and Metabolic Care*, Mar; 14(2): 121–131. DOI:10.1097/MCO.0b013e3283439622.
21. Wergin A. Mar 31, 2015. *Flaxseed is nutritionally powerful*. www.mayoclinichealthsystem.org/hometown-health/speaking-of-health/flaxseed-is-nutritionally-powerful; accessed 1/12/21.

22. Tan V. Apr 26, 2017. Top 10 health benefits of flax seeds. *Healthline*. www.healthline.com/nutrition/benefits-of-flaxseeds; accessed 1/12/21.
23. Novotny K, Fritz K, and M Parmar. No date. *Omega-3 fatty acids*. StatPearls (Internet). www.ncbi.nlm.nih.gov/books/NBK564314/ls.
24. King DE, Mainous AG, and ME Geesey. 2008. Variation in L-arginine intake follow demographics and lifestyle factors that may impact cardiovascular disease risk. *Nutrient Research*, Jan; 28(1): 21–24. DOI:10.1016/j.nutres.2007.11.003.
25. Mirmiran P, Bahadoran Z, Ghasemi A, and F Azizi. 2016. The association of dietary L-arginine intake and serum nitric oxide metabolites in adults: A population-based study. *Nutrients*, May; 8(5): 311. DOI:10.3390/nu8050311.
26. WebMD. www.webmd.com/diet/supplement-guide-l-arginine#1; accessed 1/12/21.
27. Healthline. www.healthline.com/nutrition/l-arginine; accessed 1/12/21.
28. McNeal CJ, Meininger CJ, Wilborn CD, Tekwe CD, and G Wu. 2018. Safety of dietary supplementation with arginine in adult humans. *Amino Acids*, Sep; 50(9): 1215–1229. DOI:10.1007/s00726-018-2594-7.
29. www.grandviewresearch.com/industry-analysis/flaxseeds-market; accessed 2/12/21.
30. https://badgut.org/information-centre/a-z-digestive-topics/flax-what-you-need-to-know/; accessed 3/12/21.
31. Healthline. www.healthline.com/nutrition/foods/flaxseeds; accessed 3/12/21. www.mayoclinic.org/healthy-lifestyle/nutrition-and-healthy-eating/expert-answers/flaxseed/faq-20058354; accessed 4/12/21.
32. Sargi SC, Silva BC, Santos HMC, Montanher PF, Boeing JS, Santos OO Jr, Souza NE, and JV Visentainer. 2013. Antioxidant capacity and chemical composition in seeds rich in omega-3: Chia, flax, and perilla. *Food Science and Technolology*, Sept; 33(3). DOI:10.1590/S0101-20612013005000057.
33. www.mayoclinic.org/healthy-lifestyle/nutrition-and-healthy-eating/expert-answers/flaxseed/faq-20058354; accessed 4/12/21.

2 Flaxseed, a Functional Food—Constituents and Their Health Benefits

2.1 INTRODUCTION

"Wherever flaxseeds become a regular food item among the people, there will be better health." So said Mohandas (Mahatma) Gandhi (1869–1948). Now, there's an endorsement, if ever there was one. Indeed, flaxseeds are emerging as an important functional food and food ingredient. They rank among the top 100 of the world's healthiest foods. This is largely due to rich contents of *alpha*-linolenic acid (ALA, omega-3 fatty acid), fiber and lignans. The lignans are a large group of polyphenols, dietary antioxidants found in plants that include the familiar quercetin in apples and resveratrol in red wine.

Flaxseeds, flaxseed oil, fibers and flax lignans are shown to reduce atherosclerosis, heart disease, type 2 diabetes, arthritis, osteoporosis, autoimmune and neurological disorders and cancer. Flax protein helps in the prevention and treatment of heart disease, and it supports the immune system.

Flaxseeds can be used as roasted and milled seeds, while flaxseed oil can be used in various food formulations in the form of neat oils and stable emulsions. Flax or flaxseed oil has been incorporated into baked foods, juices, milk and dairy products, muffins, dry pasta products, macaroni and beef patties.

2.2 CONSTITUENTS THAT MAKE FLAXSEED A FUNCTIONAL FOOD

Flaxseeds are available in two basic varieties: brown and yellow or golden. Both have similar nutritional characteristics and equal numbers of short-chain omega-3 fatty acids. Omega-3 fatty acids are important fats that the body needs that it must get from the diet because the body cannot produce them. The three most important types are

- Alpha-linolenic acid (ALA)
- Docosahexaenoic acid (DHA)
- Eicosapentaenoic acid (EPA)

ALA is mainly found in plants, seeds and nuts, including flaxseeds, chia seeds, flaxseed oil and walnuts. DHA and EPA occur mostly in animal foods, such as fatty fish, fish oils and algae.

TABLE 2.1
Composition of nutrient and phytochemicals in flaxseed

Nutrients/Bioactive Compounds	Quantity/100 g of Seed	Nutrients/Bioactive Compounds	Quantity/100 g of Seed
Carbohydrates	29.0 g	Biotin	6 mg
Protein	20.0 g	α-Tocopherolb	7 mg
Total fats	41.0 g	δ-Tocopherolb	10 mg
Linolenic acid	23.0 g	γ-Tocopherolb	552 mg
Dietary fiber	28.0 g	Calcium	236 mg
Lignans	10–2,600 mg	Copper	1 mg
Ascorbic acid	0.50 mg	Magnesium	431 mg
Thiamin	0.53 mg	Manganese	3 mg
Riboflavin	0.23 mg	Phosphorus	622 mg
Niacin	3.21 mg	Potassium	831 mg
Pyridoxin	0.61 mg	Sodium	27 mg
Pantothenic acid	0.57 mg	Zinc	4 mg
Folic acid	112 mg		

Source: With permission.
(2) *Journal of Food Science and Technology*. Goyal, Sharma, Upadhyay et al. 2014.

Parenthetically, in order to meet the fatty acid composition profile of the margarine industry, mutation breeding efforts led to development of flax varieties with major reductions in ALA levels (approximately 3%). These flax varieties were known as Linola™ or solin and registered and produced in Canada. The fatty acid composition of solin oil is similar to other premium polyunsaturated oils, such as sunflower oil. Oils from such varieties have higher solidification temperatures that are suitable for the margarine industry. (1)

Various edible forms of flax are available in food markets, including whole flaxseeds, milled flax, roasted flax and flax oil. Flaxseed contains many bioactive plant substances, such as oil, protein, dietary fiber, soluble polysaccharides, vitamins (A, C, F and E) and minerals (potassium, magnesium, phosphorus, sodium, iron, copper, manganese and zinc), lignans and phenolic compounds.

Phenolic compounds are ubiquitous in plants. They are an essential part of our diet and very important to us because of their antioxidant properties. Phenolic compounds include flavonoids found in foods and beverages of plant origin, such as fruits, vegetables, tea, cocoa and wine. They account for more than half of the more than 8,000 different phenolic compounds that we consume. Table 2.1 shows the composition of flaxseed.

2.3 FLAXSEED OIL/LIPIDS COMPONENTS

Flaxseed is the richest known plant source of the omega-3 fatty acid ALA. It is low in saturated fatty acids (9%), moderate in monosaturated fatty acids (18%) and rich in polyunsaturated fatty acid (73%). Of all lipids in flaxseed oil, ALA is the major

TABLE 2.2
Major fatty acids profile in flaxseed oil

Fatty Acids	Percentage (%) (Range)
Palmitic acid (C16:0)	4.90–8.00
Stearic acid (C18:0)	2.24–4.59
Oleic acid (C18:1)	13.44–19.39
Linoleic acid (C18:2) (ω-6)	12.25–17.44
α-Linolenic acid (C18:3) (ω-3)	39.90–60.42

Source: With permission.
(2) Goyal, Sharma, Upadhyay et al. 2014. *Journal of Food Science and Technology*.

fatty acid ranging from 39.00 to 60.42% followed by oleic, linoleic, palmitic and stearic acids (see Table 2.2). Flaxseed provides an excellent omega-6 to omega-3 fatty acid ratio (1:4).

Although flaxseed oil is naturally high in antioxidants like tocopherols and beta-carotene, traditional flaxseed oil easily oxidizes after being extracted and purified.

The bioavailability of ALA is dependent on the type of flax consumed. For instance, ALA has greater bioavailability in oil than in milled seed, and it has greater bioavailability in oil and milled seed than in whole seed. Table 2.2 shows the fatty acid profile in flaxseed oil.

2.4 PROTEINS

The protein content of flaxseed varies from 20% to 30% and it has an amino acid profile comparable to that of soybean, but it contains no gluten. Amino acids are organic compounds (meaning they contain carbon), with at least one nitrogen group, that combine to form proteins. Digestion breaks down amino acids just as the body uses amino acids to rebuild proteins.

Amino acids are classified into three groups:

- *Essential amino acids* cannot be made by the body, and so they must come from food. There are nine essential amino acids: histidine, isoleucine, leucine, lysine, methionine, phenylalanine, threonine, tryptophan and valine.
- *Nonessential amino acids* can be produced by the body. These are alanine, asparagine, aspartic acid, cysteine, glutamic acid, glutamine, glycine, proline, serine and tyrosine.
- *Conditional amino acids* are usually not essential, except in times of illness and stress. These are arginine, cysteine, glutamine, tyrosine, glycine, ornithine, proline and serine.

One does not need essential and nonessential amino acids at every meal, but getting a balance of them over the whole day is important. (3) Flax protein is not considered to be a complete protein due to the presence of the limiting amino acid lysine.

Whole flaxseed, flaxseed meals and isolated proteins are rich sources of glutamic acid/glutamine, L-arginine, branched-chain amino acids (valine and leucine) and aromatic amino acid (tyrosine and phenylalanine). The total nitrogen content in flaxseed is 3.25 grams/100 grams of seed.

> *Some people may have been advised to restrict their intake of the amino acid L-arginine. For instance, persons with active herpes infection, or those with Multiple myeloma or early Mm-protein markers may (should, actually) have been advised by their healthcare providers to limit their intake of L-arginine—even of foods high in contents of that amino acid. Multiple myeloma is an* auxotrophic mast-*cell mutation with a specific nutrient requirement of L-arginine caused by the loss of the ability to synthesize it. (4) In addition, persons with hyperactivated immune system response would also be well advised to limit L-arginine intake.*

The content of L-arginine is not the same in different types of flaxseed. In the basic type of flaxseed, the amount of L-arginine in 100 grams is 1.925 grams. For a typical serving size of 1 cup of whole flax seed (or 168 grams), the amount of L-arginine is 3.23 grams. (5) For persons with herpes who will be concerned, the equivalent lysine content is 1.45 grams, so they may need to supplement with extra lysine to prevent an arginine-triggered activation of the virus. By comparison, chickpeas, or garbanzo beans, contain 3.878 grams per cup, which is a much more favorable (approx. 1:1) ratio.

> *In connection with caveats concerning L-arginine, flaxseed* oil *may be the preferred supplement because it contains no L-arginine. However, flaxseeds are a* whole food *providing a host of benefits not available in flaxseed oil, the latter not being a whole food.*

2.5 DIETARY FIBER

The total flax plant is approximately 25% seeds, and 75% stem and leaves. The stem or nonseed parts are about 20% fiber, which can be extracted by chemical or mechanical retting. Retting is a process employing the action of micro-organisms and moisture on plants to dissolve or rot away much of the cellular tissues and pectins surrounding fiber bundles and so facilitating separation of the fiber from the stem.

Flax fiber is soft, lustrous and flexible; bundles of fiber have the appearance of blonde hair, hence the description "flaxen." It is stronger than cotton fiber but less elastic.

Flax fibers include both soluble and insoluble dietary fibers. The ratio of soluble to insoluble fiber varies between 20–80 and 40–60. The major insoluble fiber fraction consists of cellulose and lignin, and the soluble fiber fractions are the mucilage gums that can be extracted by water and have good foam-stabilizing properties.

Cellulose is an insoluble substance that is the main constituent of plant cell walls and of vegetable fibers, such as cotton. Lignin is a complex organic material deposited in the cell walls of many plants, making them rigid and woody.

Mucilage gums are polysaccharides that become viscous when mixed with water or other fluids and have an important role in laxatives. Polysaccharides are carbohydrates, such as starch, cellulose or glycogen, whose molecules consist of a number of sugar molecules bonded together as a polymer.

Just 10 grams of flaxseed in the daily diet increases the daily fiber intake by 1 gram of soluble fiber and by 3 grams of insoluble fiber. Insoluble fiber helps improve laxation and prevent constipation, mainly by increasing fecal bulk and reducing bowel transit time. On the other hand, water-soluble fiber helps in maintaining blood glucose levels and lowering blood cholesterol levels.

2.6 LIGNANS

Plant lignans are phenolic compounds present in almost all plants. They act as both antioxidants and phytoestrogens. Phytoestrogens can have weak estrogen activity in animals and humans. Flax contains up to 800 times more lignans than other plant foods (and their content in flaxseed is principally composed of secoisolariciresinol diglucoside (SDG) (294–700 mg/100 gram), matairesinol (0.55 mg/100 gram), lariciresinol (3.04 mg/100 gram) and pinoresinol (3.32 mg/100 g).

One source reported SDG content in the range of 11.7 to 24.1 mg/gram and 6.1 to 13.3 mg/gram in defatted flaxseed flour and whole flaxseed, respectively. (6)

Besides lignans, other phenolic compounds found in flaxseed are p-coumaric acid and ferulic acid. P-coumaric acid is a plant metabolic by-product that exhibits antioxidant and anti-inflammatory properties. It also shows bactericidal activity by damaging bacterial cell membranes and by interacting with bacterial DNA. Ferulic acid is an antioxidant that works to boost the effects of other antioxidants. It is commonly used in skin care products to protect overall skin integrity by reducing the development of fine lines, spots and wrinkles.

SDG found in flax and other foods is converted by bacteria in the gut to the lignans enterodiol and enterolactone, which can provide health benefits due to their weak estrogenic or antiestrogenic, as well as antioxidant effects. Studies have shown that largely due to its antioxidant properties, SDG offers health benefits, including protective effects against cardiovascular diseases, diabetes, cancer and mental stress. (7)

2.7 MINERALS

A 30-gram serving of flaxseed holds 7% to 30% of the recommended dietary allowances (RDAs) of calcium, magnesium and phosphorus. The approximate content of different minerals is shown in Table 2.1. Potassium content is high and comparable to those levels of recommended sources such as bananas. Potassium intake lowers the incidence of stroke, and it reduces blood platelet aggregation—often a precursor of stroke.

2.8 THE HEALTH BENEFITS OF FLAXSEED

Flaxseed bestows health benefits in addition to nutrition for five main reasons:

- First, it is high in omega-3 α-linolenic acid
- Second, it is rich in dietary soluble and insoluble fibers

- Third, due to its high content of lignans, acting as antioxidants and phytoestrogens. ALA can be metabolized in the body into DHA (omega-3) and EPA (omega-3)
- Fourth, it contains L-arginine, a NO-donor
- Fifth, it contains cyanogenic glycosides (CNglcs), a NO-donor

The health benefits of all omega-3 fatty acids (ALA, EPA and DHA) have been widely reported for several conditions, including cardiovascular disease, hypertension, atherosclerosis, diabetes, cancer, arthritis, osteoporosis, autoimmune and neurological disorders. Flaxseed has also been reported to be anti-arrhythmic, normalizing the heartbeat; anti-atherogenic, lowering the tendency to form arterial plaque; and anti-inflammatory, thereby improving blood vessel function. These benefits are schematized in Figure 2.1.

Let's take a look at some of these benefits one by one.

Flaxseed Decreases the Level of Proinflammatory Cytokines: A proinflammatory cytokine is a molecule formed by immune system cells like helper T cells and macrophages, and sent out throughout the body promoting inflammation. A study reported in the *American Journal of Clinical Nutrition* compared the effects of either flaxseed-based diets high in ALC or high in linoleic acid or an average American diet on inflammation in participants with elevated serum lipids (hypercholesterolemia).

It was found that increased consumption of dietary ALA is markedly anti-inflammatory and heart protective. (8)

Flaxseed Increases the Production of Serotonin: Neurotransmitters are often referred to as the body's chemical messengers. They are the molecules used by the nervous system to transmit messages between nerves (neurons) or from nerves to muscles.

Communication between two nerves or between nerves and muscles takes place in the small gap (synapse) between nerve fibers, or between nerve fibers and muscles, beginning as a brief electrical signal rapidly converted into a chemical neurotransmitter substance. This chemical reaction then causes a specific response in the receiving neuron or muscle downstream.

Neurotransmitters influence neurons in one of three ways:

- *Excitatory neurotransmitters* turn things ON.
- *Inhibitory transmitters* prevent things from happening. In a sense, they turn things OFF.
- *Neuromodulator neurotransmitters* operate over a slower time course than excitatory and inhibitory transmitters.

These neurotransmitter chemical molecules and their interactions are involved in countless functions of the nervous system, as well as controlling bodily functions.

Serotonin is a substance mainly found in the brain, the bowels and blood platelets. It transmits messages between nerve cells throughout the body and in the brain. Sometimes called the "happy chemical" because it contributes to our feeling of well-being and happiness, it is the precursor for melatonin that helps the body's

Flaxseed, a Functional Food

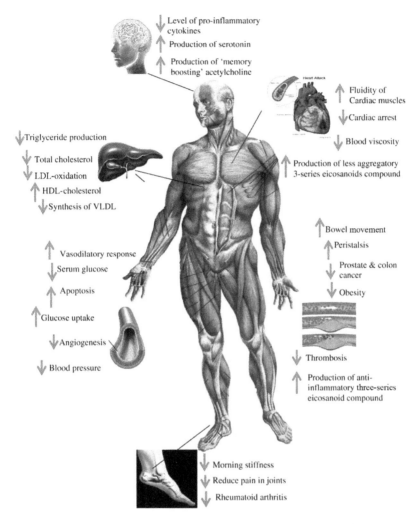

FIGURE 2.1 Health targets of the functional elements of flaxseed including oil, fiber and lignans. [(2) Goyal, Sharma, Upadhyay et al. 2014. *Journal of Food Science and Technology*. With permission.]

sleep-wake cycles and the internal clock. It also plays a role in appetite, emotions and motor, cognitive and autonomic functions.

Serotonin appears to play a key role in maintaining mood balance: Low serotonin levels have been linked to depression. In fact, a 2015 report in the journal *Clinical Psychopharmacology and Neuroscience* tells us that there is substantial clinical evidence that omega-3 polyunsaturated fatty acids (PUFAs) such as those in flaxseed may prevent mood and anxiety disorders. (9)

Flaxseed Raises the Production of "Memory Boosting" Acetylcholine: Acetylcholine (Ach) is a neurotransmitter. One of its primary functions is to carry signals from motor neurons to the skeletal muscles. It can be excitatory or inhibitory depending on the site of its action: It is excitatory at the neuromuscular junction in skeletal muscle—voluntary striated muscle—causing the muscle to contract. In contrast, it is inhibitory in blood vessels—involuntary smooth muscle—and the heart, an involuntary striated muscle—where it can lower blood pressure and slow heart rate.

The journal *Genes and Nutrition* reported in 2009 that dietary PUFAs improve cognitive function in the "aging brain" because of improved acetylcholine availability. (10) PUFAs are found in profusion in flaxseed.

Flaxseed Decreases Blood Pressure and Improves Heart Function: According to the American Heart Association (AHA): Consuming flaxseed may help lower blood pressure in people with hypertension. People who added 30 grams of milled flaxseed to their diet every day for 6 months saw their systolic blood pressure decline by an average of 15 mm Hg, and their diastolic blood pressure dropped by an average of 8 mm Hg. By comparison, people on a placebo had slightly increased systolic blood pressure, while diastolic pressure remained steady. The researchers said that the level of blood pressure decrease from adding flaxseed could result in 50% fewer strokes and 30% fewer heart attacks. (11)

Flaxseed Prevents Cardiovascular Disease: Alpha-linolenic acid (ALA), an omega-3 PUFA found in flaxseed, may reduce cardiovascular risk by regulating platelet function, reducing inflammation, enhancing endothelial cell function, raising arterial compliance (blood vessel flexibility) and reducing the risk of arrhythmia.

Modest dietary consumption of ALA (2 to 3 grams per day) is recommended for the primary and secondary prevention of cardiovascular and heart disease. (12, 13)

Flaxseed Increases Heart Muscle Lipid Fluidity: "Membrane fluidity" refers to the viscosity of the lipid in the bilayer of a cell membrane. Increasing viscosity means there is resistance to flow, causing rigidity in the membrane. Flaxseed increases the lipid fluidity of the membranes of heart muscle cells (that is, decreases rigidity), thus improving heart function. (14)

Flaxseed Reduces the Incidence of Heart Arrhythmias and the Risk of Cardiac Arrest: There is strong scientific evidence that omega-3 fatty acid supplements EPA and DHA can significantly reduce risk factors for heart disease, such as reducing blood triglyceride levels, reducing the incidence of heart arrhythmias, (15) reducing the risk of nonfatal and fatal myocardial infarctions, sudden death (13) and, by the way, reducing the risk of all-cause mortality. It should be noted, however, that, as reported in the journal *Circulation* in 2021, Smidt Heart Institute researchers have found that taking high doses of fish oil supplements EPA and DHA—specifically one gram or more per day—may increase the risk of developing atrial fibrillation. (72)

Flaxseed Decreases Blood Viscosity: Blood viscosity is the thickness and stickiness of blood affecting the ability of blood to flow. It determines the amount of work the heart has to do and the quantity of oxygen delivered to the tissues and organs. Health depends on blood flowing freely. A number of factors affect blood viscosity:

- Plasma viscosity is highly affected by hydration and by plasma proteins, especially high-molecular-weight proteins such as immunoglobulins and fibrinogen. Flaxseed was found to reduce blood plasma viscosity and fibrinogen in an animal model. (16)
- Hematocrit is the ratio of the volume of red blood cells to the total volume of blood. It is the most obvious determinant of viscosity. A higher percentage of red blood cells (RBCs) results in thicker blood. Hematocrit accounts for about 50% of the difference between normal blood viscosity and high blood viscosity. Omega-3 fatty acids in flaxseed reduce hematocrit. (17)
- Red blood cell (erythrocyte) deformability is the ability of red blood cells to change shape, i.e., to elongate and to bend and fold to pass through the slender passageways of the capillaries. The more flexible the RBCs are, the less will be the viscosity of blood, and young red blood cells are more flexible than older RBCs. Erythrocyte deformability is the second most important determinant of blood viscosity, after hematocrit. Flaxseed was found to increase RBC deformability in an animal model. (16)
- Blood platelets are a type of blood cell that helps form blood clots by sticking together (aggregation). A clot is what stops the bleeding when there is a wound. Platelet aggregation contributes to blood viscosity. Flaxseed reduces platelet aggregation. (18)

Flaxseed Promotes Healthy Bowel Function: Flaxseed's high fiber content promotes "regularity." Each one tablespoon serving of flaxseeds (about 6 grams) contains 3 grams of fiber, including a mix of both soluble and insoluble fiber. It was found to be especially helpful in persons with constipation and in those with type 2 diabetes. (19)

Flaxseed Lowers the Risk of Benign Prostate Hypertrophy: Flaxseed has been found to help maintain overall prostate health and reduce the risk of an enlarged prostate (hypertrophy), as well as lower urinary tract symptoms (LUTS). (20)

Flaxseed and Flaxseed Oil Reduces Joint Pain and Arthritis: According to the Arthritis Foundation, *Living with Arthritis* blog, just two tablespoons of ground flaxseed contain more than 140% of the daily value of the inflammation-reducing omega-3 fatty acids, and 50% of the total fatty acids in flaxseed oil is ALA, one of three omega-3 fatty acids. When consumed, ALA is converted into the other, more powerful omega-3s, DHA and EPA acids. Ground flaxseed has ALA, but flaxseed oil contains the highest amount. In a study where volunteers consumed flaxseed oil for four weeks, the ALAs significantly decreased proinflammatory compounds. (13, 21)

Flaxseed Increases Insulin Production and Reduces Blood Glucose Level: Individuals with diabetes are at increased risk of developing blood vessel complications leading to retinopathy, nephropathy, and neuropathy, in addition to cardiovascular disease (CVD). The Diabetes Control and Complications Trial (22) and UK Prospective Diabetes Study showed that flaxseed in treatment programs resulted in improved blood glucose control, as measured by HbA1c, and reduced micro-blood vessel complications of diabetes. (23)

Consuming flaxseed reduces blood sugar levels after a meal (postprandial) and increases insulin levels in prediabetic individuals. (24)

Flaxseed Improves Liver Function: Nonalcoholic fatty liver disease (NAFLD) is the buildup of extra fat in liver cells that is not caused by alcohol consumption. It is normal for the liver to contain some fat. However, if more than 5% to 10% of liver weight is fat, then it is called "fatty liver" or steatosis. It was reported in the *International Journal of Food Science and Nutrition*, in 2016, that flaxseed supplementation is effective in alleviating NAFLD. (25)

Flaxseed Improves Kidney Function: Chronic kidney disease (CKD) is an important health problem among older adults and can lead to end-stage renal disease with its need for dialysis or transplantation for survival. (26, 27)

Due to the anti-inflammatory properties of omega-3 fatty acids plentiful in flaxseed and flaxseed oil, it has been suggested that in adults, these nutrients may protect the kidneys from damage. PUFAs supplementation was observed to reduce kidney inflammation and fibrosis in animal models. (28) Increased dietary intake of long-chain omega-3 PUFA was inversely associated with the prevalence of CKD in the Blue Mountains Eye Study (1997–1999) (29).

Flaxseed Improves Lipid Profile: The lipid profile or lipid panel is a set of screening blood test results used to describe obtained blood serum levels of lipids, such as cholesterol, and triglycerides, in comparison to standard healthy values. It is used to screen for abnormalities. Serum lipid profile is directly related to the risk factors of cardiovascular diseases. It is the most intensely investigated effect studied after dietary supplementation of flaxseed or flax oil.

The journal *Reviews on Recent Clinical Trials* reported in 2015 that "flaxseed may be regarded as a useful therapeutic food for reducing hyperlipidemia," the latter meaning elevated serum cholesterol. (30) Another study published in the journal *Current Pharmaceutical Design*, in 2016, concluded that the secoisolariciresinol diglucoside (SDG) in flaxseed slows the progression of and even reverses atherosclerosis, and that it could serve as an alternative medicine for the treatment of coronary artery disease, stroke and peripheral arterial vascular diseases. (31)

Flaxseed Improves Health Hazards of Menopause: A study published in the journal *Holistic Nursing Practice*, in 2015, reported on the effects of flaxseed on menopausal symptoms and quality of life throughout the menopausal period. The empirical research was conducted in the obstetrics and gynecology outpatient department of a university hospital in Izmir, Turkey. The menopausal symptoms decreased, and the quality of life increased among the women who used flaxseed for three months. (32)

2.9 CNglcs IN FLAXSEEDS, NO-DONORS

According to a report in the *Journal of Agricultural and Food Chemistry*, CNglcs are nitrogenous secondary metabolites derived from amino acids. There are several major categories, including linustatin and neolinustatin, a β-gentiobioside of acetone cyanohydrin and methyl ethyl ketone cyanohydrins. There are also minor components, including linamarin (1-cyano-1-methylethyl β-D-glycopyranoside), along with diglucosides linustatin and neolinustatin. The quantity of constituents found in various cultivars has, however, been shown to vary from sample to sample tested, depending also on seasonal effect and on the location where they were grown. (33)

In fact, the journal *Food and Nutrition Sciences* reported on the content of the CNglcs (linamarin, linustatin and neolinustatin) in 21 varieties belonging to different groups producing oil, fiber and intermediate products. The total content of CNglcs ranged from 0.74 to 1.60 g • Kg^{-1} CN^{-1}. As expected, linamarin was a minor component, accounting for only about 2% of total glycosides.

Linustatin was significantly lower in the intermediate group than in the other groups, and, in particular, it was the lowest in the Festival variety. Neolinustatin was lower in the fiber group, although the variety Ventimiglia (belonging to the oil group) showed a negligible level of this compound. Neolinustatin was positively correlated to total CNglcs and inversely correlated to linustatin. (34)

2.10 GUIDELINES TO SUPPLEMENTATION OF FLAXSEED AND FLAXSEED OIL

According to SELFNutritionData, Nutrition Facts, a typical serving size of ground flaxseeds is 1 tablespoon (7 grams) and it contains the following:

- Calories: 37
- Total fat: 3 grams
- Saturated fat: 0.3 grams
- Cholesterol: 0 mg
- Sodium: 2 mg
- Total carbohydrates: 2 grams
- Dietary fiber: 2 grams
- Sugar: 0 grams
- Protein: 1 gram
- Monounsaturated fat: 0.5 grams
- Polyunsaturated fat: 2.0 grams
- Omega-3 fatty acids: 1,597 mg
- Vitamin B1: 8% of the recommended daily intake (RDI)
- Vitamin B6: 2% of the RDI
- Folate: 2% of the RDI
- Calcium: 2% of the RDI
- Iron: 2% of the RDI
- Magnesium: 7% of the RDI
- Phosphorus: 4% of the RDI
- Potassium: 2% of the RDI (35)

The Mayo Clinic website reports the following:

> Flaxseed can be used whole or crushed, or in a powder form as meal or flour. Flaxseed oil is available in liquid and capsule form. People use flaxseed and flaxseed oil to

reduce cholesterol and blood sugar and treat digestive conditions. Some people also take flaxseed to treat inflammatory diseases. When used in combination with daily exercise and a low cholesterol diet, flaxseed might help control cholesterol levels. Flaxseed might also be helpful for managing diabetes and lowering the risk of heart disease.

The website of the *Institut de Montreal* features an article titled "The Positive Effects of Flaxseed on Cardiovascular Health." The author, Martin Juneau, MD, reports the recommendation of an average daily intake of 2.2 g of linolenic acid. This is said to correspond to 1 tablespoon (15 mL) of flaxseed. He further recommends grinding the seeds to raise the absorption of omega-3 fatty acids and allow the transformation of lignans into active phytoestrogens by intestinal bacteria. However, omega-3 fatty acids are very fragile and sensitive to degradation, and one should buy whole seeds that can be ground when needed in a simple coffee grinder and store the ground seeds for a maximum of two weeks in the refrigerator in an airtight container (https://observatoireprevention.org/en/2018/01/25/the-positive-effects-of-flaxseed-on-cardiovascular-health/).

When taken in recommended amounts, flaxseed and flaxseed oil are generally safe to use. However, when taken in large amounts and with too little water, flaxseed can cause bloating, gas, even diarrhea. It is best to follow these guidelines:

- Avoid use of flaxseed and flaxseed oil during pregnancy.
- Occasionally, using flaxseed or flaxseed oil causes an allergic reaction.
- Don't eat raw or unripe flaxseeds.
- Because flaxseed oil might decrease blood clotting, stop using flaxseed oil two weeks before having elective surgery.

Flaxseed supplementation may entail possible interactions, including the following:

- *Anticoagulant and anti-platelet drugs, herbs and supplements*: These types of drugs, herbs and supplements reduce blood clotting. Flaxseed oil also might decrease blood clotting. It's possible that taking flaxseed oil along with those blood-thinning agents might increase the risk of bleeding.
- *Blood pressure drugs, herbs and supplements*: Flaxseed oil might lower blood pressure. Taking flaxseed oil with drugs, herbs and supplements that lower blood pressure might lower blood pressure too much.
- *Diabetes drugs*: Flaxseed might lower blood sugar levels. Taking flaxseed with diabetes drugs or herbs or supplements with hypoglycemic potential might lower blood sugar too much.
- *Estrogens*: Flaxseed might have an anti-estrogen effect. Taking flaxseed might decrease the effects of oral contraceptive drugs and estrogen replacement therapy.
- *Oral drugs*: Taking flaxseed might decrease absorption of oral drugs. Consider taking oral drugs and flaxseed an hour or two apart. (36)

The Mayo Clinic website does not report how much one should take each day for effective supplementation, nor does it report how much is too much. There is no set

Flaxseed, a Functional Food   37

dose of flaxseed. In studies of people with high cholesterol, 15 to 50 grams of flaxseed per day has been used; 40 grams/day has been used for mild menopause symptoms.

Flaxseed must be ground prior to consumption, or it won't work for these conditions. It can be mixed with liquid or food, such as muffins or bread. But to be better absorbed, it must be ground before using it to allow the oils to be available. Some people use a small coffee grinder to grind daily doses as needed. (37)

A number of such grinders are commercially available:

- *Cool Knight brand* (manual or electric): Herb Grinder Electric Spice Grinder Spices and Herbs
- *Turimon brand*: Large Herbal Grinders/Mill/(electric): Crusher for Spice and Herbs
- *Cuisinart brand*: *Grinder—(Electric) Spice-and-Nut Grinder*
- *MotorGenic brand*: Herb Grain Grinder 700 g Electric Mill Cereal Machine
- *Prima Cucina brand*: Electric Pepper Mill With Light and Rounded Top

2.10.1 Recommended Flaxseed Supplements Content of ALA

The *Journal of Food Science and Technology* reported in 2014 that for optimal health, many governments and public health authorities recommend increasing omega-3 fatty acids in the diet. In fact, as early as 1990, Health Canada recommended an omega-6 to omega-3 fatty acid dietary ratio in the range of 4:1 to 10:1. (38)

A number of sources recommend that supplement products need to contain an amount and type of flaxseed that will significantly increase the levels of ALA in the blood over and above the recommended daily amount of 1.6 grams/day for men and 1.1 grams/day for women. (39, 40) But according to the US Department of Agriculture (USDA), flaxseed contains approximately 23 grams of ALA per 100 grams (41), and thus the recommended dietary amounts can be obtained by consuming about 9 grams of flaxseed per day. But supplement products for clinical trials need to contain sufficient flaxseed to significantly raise the levels of ALA in the blood above the recommended daily amount of 1.6 grams/day for men and 1.1 grams/day for women. (42, 43)

2.11 POTENTIAL ANTI-NUTRITIONAL ASPECTS OF FLAXSEED

Despite its health benefits, flaxseed is not totally free of constituents considered anti-nutritional, such as CNglcs. Flaxseed contains CNglcs and linamarin (acetone—cyanohydrin-beta—glucoside $C_{10}H_{17}O_6N$) in small amounts. (44) Whole flaxseed contains 250 to 550 mg of CNglcs per 100 grams, (45) of which linustatin and neolinustatin are the major components. There is reportedly about 174 to 207 mg/100 grams of linustatin and neolinustatin, respectively, in flaxseed. (46)

Damaging the seeds causes the release of β-glucosidases, contributing to the formation of hydrogen cyanide. However, adequate processing of foodstuffs containing CNglcs helps in reducing the potential risks associated with poisoning. (47, 48) For example, more than 85% of linustatin, neolinustatin, were removed when flaxseed was heated for more than two hours at 200 °C (392 °F). (46)

Flaxseed meal also contains 2.3% to 3.3% phytic acid. Phytic acid is found in nuts, edible seeds, and beans/legumes. It is the main storage form of phosphorous, and it also binds to positively charged metals, thus binding avidly to the kinds of minerals that are crucial for nutrition such as magnesium, iron and zinc, thus impairing the absorption of these minerals in the digestive tract. (49) For this reason, some health authorities advise restricting consumption of nuts, beans, grains and legumes, which are high in phytic acid, because phytic acid binds with minerals thereby potentially jeopardizing bone health. On the other hand, phytic acid has antioxidant, anticancer, hypocholesterolemic and hypolipidemic properties. (45)

Flaxseed meal also contains 10 mg/100 gram Linatine (gammaglutamyl- 1-amino-D-proline), a vitamin B6 antagonist that can induce deficiency. (45) Pyridoxal 5′-phosphate (P-5-P), a cofactor of Vitamin B-6, has a crucial role in amino acid metabolism. A prevalence of moderate vitamin B-6 deficiency in the population has been reported, and it is thought to result from the ingestion of 1-amino D-proline (1ADP) (linatine) found in flaxseed. (50) However, other investigators reported that the linatine in flaxseed did not affect vitamin B6 levels or metabolism in people fed up to 50 grams of ground flaxseed per day. (51, 52) It has also been reported that large amounts of flaxseed depressed vitamin E levels in an animal model. (51)

2.12 HEALTH BENEFITS OF FLAX PROTEINS

Flax is not commonly used as a source of food protein for humans but is used in animal feed. However, recent reports have shown it to have a number of healthful properties (53–56):

- Flaxseed proteins were shown to be beneficial in coronary heart disease, kidney disease and cancer. (57–59) For example, peptides derived from enzymatic hydrolysis of flaxseed proteins inhibited angiotensin I—converting enzyme (ACE) activities and also displayed *in vitro* antioxidant activities. (60, 61)
- Flax proteins contain significant amounts of L-arginine and glutamine (62), which are very important in the prevention and treatment of heart disease. (63)
- Peptide mixture from flaxseed with high levels of branched-chain amino acids, and low levels of aromatic amino acids have shown antioxidant properties by scavenging 2,2-diphenyl-1-picrylhydrazyl radical and antihypertensive properties by inhibiting the ACE activity. (64)
- Flaxseed supports immune system function. (65) They contain bioactive peptides such as cyclolinopeptide A, which support immune function and antimalarial activities, inhibiting the human malarial parasite *Plasmodium falciparum* in culture. (66)

Table 2.3 lists the principal biological/functional properties of flaxseed proteins and identifies the characteristics of flaxseed that make it a functional food. In particular, flaxseed supplies high levels of ALA and omega-3 fatty acids. These antioxidant constituents are well-known to the health and nutrition professions for their role in preventing—even treating—cardiovascular and heart disease, stroke, kidney failure and the symptoms of diabetes complications.

TABLE 2.3
Principal biological/functional properties of flaxseed proteins

Function of Flax Protein	Effects/Mechanism	Reference
Antifungal	Acts against food spoilage fungi *Penicilliumchrysogenum*, *Fusariumgraminearum* and *Aspergillusflavus*	67, 68
Antioxidant	Hydrolyzed flaxseed proteins exhibited antioxidant properties by scavenging 2, 2-diphenyl-1- picrylhydrazyl radical, superoxide radical and hydroxyl radical	68, 69
Antihypertensive	Inhibits angiotensin I-converting enzyme	64
Cholesterol-lowering effect	Due to their bile acid binding activity	61
Antidiabetic	Because flax proteins can interact with fiber and mucilage and also by stimulating the secretion of insulin	70
Anti-thrombic	Flax proteins- hirudine and linusitin	71
Anti-tumor	Due to presence of low lysine/arginine ratio	70

Source: With permission.
(2) Goyal, Sharma, Upadhyay et al. 2014. *Journal of Food Science and Technology*.

So far, CNglcs have only been briefly described as a constituent of flaxseed, and no detailed mention of it has been made in connection with its potential to ward off health hazards. As previously noted, that potential rests in their being an excellent and plentiful source of NO.

2.13 SUMMARY

Flaxseed, an excellent nutrient supplement, is the richest plant source of the omega-3 fatty acid ALA. It is low in saturated fatty acids (9%), moderate in monosaturated fatty acids (18%) and rich in polyunsaturated fatty acids. It is also high in fiber and in lignans, phenolic compounds that act as both antioxidants and phytoestrogens. Flaxseed contributes minerals such as calcium, magnesium and phosphorus, and it contains CNglcs, powerful NO-donors. Health benefits include reduced risk of hypertension, cardiovascular disease, atherosclerosis, diabetes, kidney failure, cancer, arthritis joint pain, osteoporosis, autoimmune and neurological disorders. Flaxseed has also been reported to be anti-arrhythmic, normalizing the heartbeat; anti-atherogenic, lowering the tendency to form arterial plaque; and anti-inflammatory, thereby improving blood vessel function. Dietary supplementation is described and very rare but potentially adverse side effects are cited.

2.14 REFERENCES

1. https://flaxcouncil.ca/growing-flax/chapters/varieties/; accessed 1/7/20.
2. Goyal A, Sharma V, Upadhyay N, Gill S, and M Sihag. 2014. Flax and flaxseed oil: An ancient medicine and modern functional food. *Journal of Food Science and Technology*, Sep; 51(9): 1633–1653. DOI:10.1007/s13197-013-1247-9.

3. https://medlineplus.gov/ency/article/002222.htm; accessed 9/10/19
4. Riess C, Shokraie F, Classen CF, Kreikemeyer B, Fiedler T, Junghanss C, and C Maletzki. 2018. Arginine-depleting enzymes—an increasingly recognized treatment strategy for therapy-refractory malignancies. *Cellular Physiology and Biochemistry*, 51: 854–870. DOI:10.1159/000495382.
5. www.dietandfitnesstoday.com/arginine-in-flaxseed.php; accessed 9/9/19.
6. Johnsson P, Kamal-Eldin A, Lundgren LN, and P Aman. 2000. HPLC method for analysis of secoisolariciresinol diglucoside in flaxseeds. *Journal of Agricultural and Food Chemistry*, Nov; 48(11): 5216–5219. DOI:10.1021/jf0005871.
7. Kezimana P, Dmitriev AA, Kudryavtseva AV, Romanova EV, and NV Melnikova. 2018. Secoisolariciresinol diglucoside of flaxseed and its metabolites: Biosynthesis and potential for nutraceuticals. *Frontiers in Genetics*, Dec 12; 9: 641. https://doi.org/10.3389/fgene.2018.00641.
8. Zhao G, Etherton TD, Martin KR, Gillies PJ, West SG, and PM Kris-Etherton. 2007. Dietary α-linolenic acid inhibits proinflammatory cytokine production by peripheral blood mononuclear cells in hypercholesterolemic subjects. *American Journal of Clinical Nutrition*, Feb; 85(20): 385–391. DOI:10.1093/ajcn/85.2.385.
9. Su K-P, Matsuoka Y, and C-U Pae. 2015. Omega-3 polyunsaturated fatty acids in prevention of mood and anxiety disorders. *Clinical Psychopharmacology and Neuroscience*, Aug; 13(2): 129–137. DOI:10.9758/cpn.2015.13.2.129.
10. Willis LM, Shukitt-Hale B, and JA Joseph. 2009. Dietary polyunsaturated fatty acids improve cholinergic transmission in the aged brain. *Genes and Nutrition*, Dec; 4(4): 309–314. DOI:10.1007/s12263-009-0141-6.
11. Eating Flaxseed May Lower Blood Pressure. www.heart.org/HEARTORG/News/News Releases/Eating-flaxseed-may-lower-blood-pressure_UCM_446258_Article.jsp#.XYUN juTsbcs; accessed 9/20/19.
12. Mozaffarian D. 2005. Does alpha-linolenic acid intake reduce the risk of coronary heart disease? A review of the evidence. *Alternative Therapies in Health and Medicine*, May–Jun; 11(3): 24–30.
13. Rodriguez-Leyva D, Bassett CMC, McCullough R, and GN Pierce. 2010. The cardiovascular effects of flaxseed and its omega-3 fatty acid, alpha-linolenic acid. *Canadian Journal of Cardiology*, Nov; 26(9): 489–496. PMCID: PMC2989356.
14. Jump DB, Depner CM, and S Tripathy. 2012. Omega-3 fatty acid supplementation and cardiovascular disease. Thematic Review Series: New lipid and lipoprotein targets for the treatment of cardiometabolic diseases. *Journal of Lipid Research*, Dec; 53(12): 2525–2545. DOI:10.1194/jlr.R027904.
15. Albert CM, Oh K, Whang W, Manson JE, Chae CU, Stampfer MJ, Willett WC, and FB Hu. 2005. Dietary alpha-linolenic acid intake and risk of sudden cardiac death and coronary heart disease. *Circulation*, Nov 22; 112(21): 3232–3238. DOI:10.1161/CIRCULATIONAHA.105.572008.
16. Anishchenko AM, Vasil'eva NV, Plotnikova TM, and OI Aliev. 2011. Effects of flaxseed extract on rheological properties of blood in experimental ovariectomy. *Eksperimental'naia i Klinicheskaia Farmakologiia*, 74(7): 19–21.
17. Ernst E. 1991. Blood fluidity and omega-3 fatty acids. *Wiener Medizinische Wochenschrift*, 141(7): 141–143.
18. Bierenbaum ML, Reichstein R, and KL Jordan. 1993. Reducing atherogenic risk in hyperlipemic humans with flax seed supplementation: A preliminary report. *Journal of the American College of Nutrition*, Aug; 12(5): 501–504. DOI:10.1080/07315724.1993.10718342.
19. Soltanian N, and M Janghorbani. 2018. A randomized trial of the effects of flaxseed to manage constipation, weight, glycemia, and lipids in constipated patients with type 2 diabetes. *Nutrition and Metabolism* (Lond), May; 15: 36. DOI:10.1186/s12986-018-0273-z.

20. Zhang W, Wang X, Liu Y, Tian H, Flickinger B, Empie MW, and SZ Sun. 2008. Effects of dietary flaxseed lignan extract on symptoms of benign prostatic hyperplasia. *Journal of Medicinal Food*, Jun; 11(2): 207–214. DOI:10.1089/jmf.2007.602.
21. http://blog.arthritis.org/living-with-arthritis/health-benefits-flaxseed-anti-inflammatory/; accessed 10/13/19.
22. Nathan DM, Genuth S, Lachin J, Cleary P, Crofford O, Davis M, Rand L, and C Siebert. 1993. The effect of intensive treatment of diabetes on the development and progression of long-term complications in insulin-dependent diabetes mellitus. *Diabetes Control and Complications Trial Research Group. NEJM*, Sep 30; 329(14): 977–986. DOI:10.1056/NEJM199309303291401.
23. Reichard P, Nilsson BY, and U Rosenqvist. 1993. The effect of long-term intensified insulin treatment on the development of microvascular complications of diabetes mellitus. *NEJM*, Jul 9; 329(5): 304–309. DOI:10.1056/NEJM199307293290502.
24. Javidi A, Mozaffari-Khosravi H, Nadjarzadeh A, Dehghani A, and MH Eftekhari. 2016. The effect of flaxseed powder on insulin resistance indices and blood pressure in prediabetic individuals: A randomized controlled clinical trial. *Journal of Research in Medical Sciences*, 21: 70. DOI:10.4103/1735-1995.189660.
25. Yari Z, Rahimlou M, Eslamparast T, Ebrahimi-Daryani N, Poustchi H, and A Hekmatdoost. 2016. Flaxseed supplementation in non-alcoholic fatty liver disease: A pilot randomized, open labeled, controlled study. *International Journal of Food Science and Nutrition*, Jun; 67(4): 461–469. DOI:10.3109/09637486.2016.1161011.
26. Coresh J, Selvin E, Stevens LA, Manzi J, Kusek JW, Eggers P, Van Lente F, and AS Levey. 2007. Prevalence of chronic kidney disease in the United States. *Journal of the American Medical Association*, Nov 7; 298(17): 2038–2047. DOI:10.1001/jama.298.17.2038.
27. Lauretani F, Maggio M, Pizzarelli F, Michelassi S, Ruggiero C, Ceda GP, Bandinelli S, and L Ferrucci. 2009. Omega-3 and renal function in older adults. *Current Pharmaceutical Design*, 15(36): 4149–4156. DOI:10.2174/138161209789909719.
28. Baggio B, Musacchio E, and G Priante. 2005. Polyunsaturated fatty acids and renal fibrosis: Pathophysiologic link and potential clinical implications. *Journal of Nephrology*, 18: 362–367.
29. Gopinath B, Harris DC, Flood VM, Burlutsky G, and P Mitchell. 2011. Consumption of long-chain n-3 PUFA, a-linolenic acid and fish is associated with the prevalence of chronic kidney disease. *British Journal of Nutrition*, May; 105(9): 1361–1368. DOI:10.1017/S0007114510005040.
30. Torkan M, Entezari MH, and M Siavash. 2015. Effect of flaxseed on blood lipid level in hyperlipidemic patients. *Reviews on Recent Clinical Trials*, 10(1): 61–67. DOI:10.2174/1574887110666150121154334.
31. Prasad K, and A Jadhav. 2016. Prevention and treatment of atherosclerosis with flaxseed-derived compound secoisolariciresinol diglucoside. *Current Pharmaceutical Design*, 22(2): 214–220. DOI:10.2174/1381612822666151112151130.
32. Cetisli NE, Saruhan A, and B Kivcak. 2015. The effects of flaxseed on menopausal symptoms and quality of life. *Holistic Nursing Practice*, May–Jun; 29(3): 151–157. DOI:10.1097/HNP.0000000000000085.
33. Oomah BD, Mazza G, and EO Kenaschuk. 1992. Cyanogenic compounds in flaxseed. *Journal of Agricultural and Food Chemistry*, Aug 1; 40(8): 1346–1348. DOI:10.1021/jf00020a010.
34. Russo R, and R Reggiani. 2014. Variation in the content of cyanogenic glycosides in flaxseed meal from twenty-one varieties. *Food and Nutrition Sciences*, Jul; 5(5): 1456–1462. DOI:10.4236/fns.2014.515159.
35. https://nutritiondata.self.com/facts/nut-and-seed-products/3163/2; accessed 10/19/19.
36. www.mayoclinic.org/drugs-supplements-flaxseed-and-flaxseed-oil/art-20366457; accessed 10/19/19.
37. www.webmd.com/a-to-z-guides/supplement-guide-flaxseed-oil#1; accessed 10/19/19.

38. No authors. 1990. Nutrition recommendation. The report of the scientific review committee. *Department of Supply and Services*. Cat. No. H49–42/1990E. Health and Welfare Canada. Ottawa, Ontario.
39. No authors. 2009. *Do Canadian adults meet their nutrient requirements through food intake alone?* www.hc-sc.gc.ca/fn-an/alt_formats/pdf/surveill/nutrition/commun/art-nutr-adult-eng.pdf; accessed 1/12/20.
40. No authors. 2010. *U. S. department of agriculture, agricultural research service, nutrient data laboratory (2010) USDA national nutrient database for standard reference, release 23.* www.nal.usda.gov/fnic/usda-nutrient-data-laboratory; accessed 1/12/20.
41. No authors. 2010a. *USDA Dietary guidelines for Americans.* U.S. Department of Agriculture. U.S. Dept. of Health and Human Services. https://health.gov/dietaryguidelines/dga2010/dietaryguidelines2010.pdf; accessed 10/22/19. DOI:10.1021/jf00020a010.
42. Website ref. 2.10: Health Canada. 2009. *Do Canadian adults meet their nutrient requirements through food intake alone?* www.canada.ca/en/health-canada/services/food-nutrition/food-nutrition-surveillance/health-nutrition-surveys/canadian-community-health-survey-cchs/canadian-adults-meet-their-nutrient-requirements-through-food-intake-alone-health-canada-2012.html; accessed 1/12/19.
43. No authors. 2010b. *Composition of foods raw, processed, prepared USDA national nutrient database for standard reference, release 23.* www.ars.usda.gov/ARSUserFiles/80400525/Data/SR23/sr23_doc.pdf; accessed 1/12/20.
44. Hall C, Tulbek MC, and Y Xu. 2006. Flaxseed. *Advances in Food and Nutrition Research*, 51: 1–97. DOI:10.1016/S1043-4526(06)51001-0.
45. Mazza G. 2008. *Production, processing and uses of Canadian flax.* First CGNA International Workshop, Temuco, Chile, Aug 3–6.
46. Park ER, Hong JH, Lee DH, Han SB, Lee KB, Park JS, Chung HW, Hong KH, and MC Kim. 2005. Analysis and decrease of cyanogenic glucosides in flaxseed. *Journal of the Korean Society of Food Science and Nutrition*, 34: 875–879. DOI:10.3746/jkfn.2005.34.6.875.
47. Ernesto M, Cardoso AP, Nicala D, Mirione E, Massaza F, Cliff J, Haque MR, and JH Bradbury. 2002. Persistent konzo and cyanogen toxicity from cassava in northern Mozambique. *Acta Tropica*, 82: 357–362.
48. Haque RM, and JH Bradbury. 2002. Total cyanide determination of plants and foods using the picrate and acid hydrolysis methods. *Food Chemistry*, 77: 107–114. DOI:10.1016/S0308-8146(01)00313-2.
49. www.menshealth.com/health/a20914315/what-is-phytic-acid/.
50. Mayengbam S, Raposo S, Aliani M, and JD House. 2016. A vitamin B-6 antagonist from flaxseed perturbs amino acid metabolism in moderately vitamin B-6—deficient male rats. *The Journal of Nutrition*, Jan; 146(1): 14–20. DOI:10.3945/jn.115.219378.
51. Ratnayake WMN, Behrens WA, Fischer PWF, Labbe MR, Mongeau R, and JL Beare-Rogers. 1992. Flaxseed, chemical stability and nutritional properties. *Proceedings of the Flax Institute, US*, 54: 37.
52. Dieken HA. 1992. Use of flaxseed as a source of omega-3 fatty acids in human nutrition. In *The 54th Proceeding of the Flax Institute*. US, pp. 1–4.
53. Wang B, Dong L, Wang LJ, and N Ozkan. 2010. Effect of concentrated flaxseed protein on the solubility and rheological properties of soybean oil-in-water emulsions. *Journal of Food Engineering*, 96: 555–561.
54. Mueller K, Eisner P, and E Kirchhoff. 2010. Simplified fractionation process for linseed meal by alkaline extraction-functional properties of protein and fiber fractions. *Journal of Food Engineering*, 99: 49–54.
55. Mueller K, Eisner P, Yoshie-Stark Y, Nakada R, and E Kirchhoff. 2010. Functional properties and chemical composition of fractionated brown and yellow linseed meal (*Linum usitatissimum* L.). *Journal of Food Engineering*, 98: 453–460.

56. Green BE, Martens R, Tergesen J, and R Milanova. 2005. *Flax protein isolates and production*. US patent 2005/0107593 A1.
57. Oomah BD, and G Mazza. 2000. Bioactive components of flaxseed: Occurrence and health benefits. In: Shahidi F, and CT Ho, eds. *Phytochemicals and phytopharmaceuticals*. Champaign: AOCS Press, pp. 105–120.
58. Wang B, Li D, Wang LJ, Huang ZG, Zhang L, Chen XD, and ZH Mao. 2007. Effect of moisture content on the physical properties of fibered flaxseed. *International Journal of Food Engineering*, 3: 1–11.
59. Wang B, Wang LJ, Li D, Bhandari B, Wu WF, Shi J, Chen XD, and Zh Mao. 2009. Effects of potato starch addition and cooling rate on rheological characteristics of flaxseed protein concentrate. *Journal of Food Engineering*, 3: 392–401.
60. Omoni AO, and RE Aluko. 2006. Effect of cationic flaxseed protein hydrolysate fractions on the in vitro structure and activity of calmodulin-dependent endothelial nitric oxide synthase. *Molecular Nutrition and Food Research*, 50: 958–966. DOI:10.1002/mnfr.200600041.
61. Marambe PWMLHK, Shand PJ, and JPD Wanasundara. 2008. An in vitro investigation of selected biological activities of hydrolyzed flaxseed (*Linum usitatissimum* L.) proteins. *Journal of the American Oil Chemists' Society*, 85: 1155–1164. DOI:10.107/s11746-008-1293-z.
62. Oomah BD, and G Mazza. 1993. Flaxseed proteins—A review. *Food Chemistry*, 48: 109–114.
63. Gornik HL, and MA Creager. 2004. Arginine and endothelial and vascular health. *Journal of Nutrition*, 134(10): 2880S–2887S.
64. Udenigwe CC, and RE Aluko. 2010. Antioxidant and angiotensin converting enzyme-inhibitory properties of a flaxseed protein-derived high Fischer ratio peptide mixture. *Journal of Agricultural and Food Chemistry*, Apr 28; 58(8): 4762–4768. DOI:10.1021/jf100149w.
65. Avenell A. 2006. Glutamine in critical care: Current evidence from systematic reviews. *Proceedings of the Nutrition Society*, Aug; 65(3): 236–241. DOI:10.1079/pns2006498.
66. Bell A, McSteen PM, Cebrat M, Picur B, and IZ Siemion. 2000. Antimalarial activity of cyclolinopeptide A and its analogues. *Acta Pololoniea Pharmaceutica*, Nov; 57(Suppl): 134–136.
67. Xu Y, Hall C, Wolf-Hall C, and F Manthey. 2006. Antifungal activity of flaxseed flours. In: Carter JF, ed. *Proocedings of the 61st Flax Institute of the U.S*. Fargo: North Dakota State University, pp. 177–185.
68. Xu Y, Hall IIC, and C Wolf-Hall. 2008. Antifungal activity stability of flaxseed protein extracts using response surface methodology. *Journal of Food Science*, 73: M9–M14.
69. Udenigwea CC, Lub YL, Hanb CH, Houc WC, and RE Aluko. 2009. Flaxseed protein-derived peptide fractions: Antioxidant properties and inhibition of lipopolysaccharide-induced nitric oxide production in murine macrophages. *Food Chemistry*, 116(1): 277–284.
70. Oomah BD. 2001. Flaxseed as a functional food source. *Journal of the Science of Food and Agriculture*, 81(9): 889–894.
71. Tolkachev ON, and AA Zhuchenko. 2000. Biologically active substances of flax: Medicinal and nutritional properties (a review). *Pharmaceutical Chemistry Journal*, 34(7): 360–367.
72. Gencer B, Djousse L, Al-Ramady OT, Cook NR, Manson JE, and CM Albert. 2021. Effect of long-term marine ω-3 fatty acids supplementation on the risk of atrial fibrillation in randomized controlled trials of cardiovascular outcomes: A systematic review and meta-analysis. *Circulation*, 144(25): 1981–1990. DOI:10.1161/circulationaha.121.055654.

3 The Beneficial Effect of Omega-3 PUFA and L-Arginine on Endothelial Nitric Oxide (NO) Bioavailability

3.1 THE MORE YOU NO

This chapter will first review aspects of the basic structure and physiology of arterial blood vessels and their control systems. Then it will detail the contribution of constituents of flaxseed, i.e., omega-3 PUFAs and L-arginine, to maintaining their healthy function.

All our cells, tissues and organs depend on oxygen (O_2) supplied by blood. And the heart that *helps keep* blood flowing under pressure to our cells, tissues and organs likewise depends on a reliable oxygen-rich blood supply. Blood flow is under the control of a number of factors and principal among them is *tonus*—degree of constriction—regulated to a significant extent by the biological formation of a gas, endothelial nitric oxide (eNO).

We italicized "*helps keep*" to emphasize that the conventional notion that blood circulates under the action of the heart as a pump within vessels that can only constrict or dilate is *reductio ad absurdum*. Blood actually flows under the active pumping control of virtually all segments of the circulatory system once it leaves the heart.

As noted in previous chapters, flax contributes many of its constituents to maintaining blood vessel and heart health, and two of the most important are L-arginine and the cyanogenic glycosides (CNglcs) because both of these form that key component of blood vessel modulation and heart function, the gas molecule nitric oxide (NO), as you will see. It was also briefly noted previously that it was discovered in the early 1980s that a substance essential to healthy blood circulation, the gas NO, ordinarily formed in the body from the amino acid L-arginine, can also be formed by digestive enzymes from the CNglcs in certain foodstuffs, notably flaxseed.

CNglcs are considered natural plant "toxins" that are present in minute quantities in a number of plants, most of which we consume. It is thought that they are part of the plant defenses against insects, microbes and certain other predators. Their toxicity derives from the fact that when digested, they can release minute quantities of cyanide, which, as noted in previous chapters, is harmless to people at low doses. Cyanide can be chemically decomposed in the body to yield NO. In fact, sodium nitroprusside is a NO-based drug that is used for vasodilation in emergency settings to treat acute hypertension. (46)

The body commonly forms NO from the amino acid L-arginine found in high concentrations in meats, protein-rich legumes and nuts and in foods rich in nitrates. Flaxseed holding CNglcs, a source of NO, therefore makes it a useful nutrient supplement in general to enhance NO availability and a valuable alternative to the amino acid L-arginine as a source of NO, especially where an arginine-deprivation diet is recommended.

There is, by the way, no appreciable amounts of CNglcs in flaxseed oil.

NO regulates blood flow by triggering a cascade of events that result in relaxation of arterial vessel smooth muscle. Absent NO, blood vessels, the heart and the kidneys falter. And, as will be shown, by the way, so do the nervous system and the immune system falter.

It is very important, therefore, to know what NO is, how it is formed and especially what it does in the body to appreciate the contribution of flaxseed as a NO-donor supplement. This chapter will address these issues, and the following chapters will then detail the role of NO, the consequences of NO unavailability and the efficacy of increasing NO availability in a number of our unfortunately all too common health hazards.

3.2 NITRIC OXIDE: THE 1992 *SCIENCE* "MOLECULE OF THE YEAR"

In 1992, the prestigious journal *Science* took the very unusual step of declaring nitric oxide (NO) the *Molecule of the Year*. Biological and medical scientists were at first in utter disbelief that a gas could play a crucial biological regulatory role in the body. But today, searching "nitric oxide" on the US National Library of Medicine website (PubMed) would result in more than 226,939 medical science journal title entries linking it to virtually every known health condition, including asthma, cardiovascular and heart disease, diabetes, kidney failure, toxemia of pregnancy, cancer, sickle cell disease, erectile dysfunction and many more. Here is a small sample:

- NO lowers blood pressure (Bode-Böger, Böger, Creutzig et al. 1994: *Clinical Science*, 87; 303–310).
- NO reduces the workload of the heart (Rector, Bank, Mullen et al. 1996: *Circulation*, 93; 2135–2141).
- NO is antioxidant at low concentrations (Wolf, Zalpour, Theilmeier et al. 1997: *Journal of the American College of Cardiology*, 29; 479–485).
- NO regulates kidney function (Mount and Power. 2006. *Acta Physiologica* (Oxf), Aug; 187(4): 433–446).
- *NO reduces insulin resista*nce in type-2 diabetes (Piatti, Monti, Valsecchi et al. 2001. *Diabetes Care*, 24; 875–880).
- NO ameliorates sickle cell disease (Reiter and Gladwin. 2003. *Current Opinion in Hematology*, Mar; 10(2): 99–107).
- NO strengthens penile erection (Zorgniotti and Lizza 1994: *International Journal of Impotence Research*, 6; 33–35).

Clearly, it is highly desirable to maintain NO availability throughout our life span, but unfortunately, we normally gradually lose the ability to form it as we age. (1) However, we can increase NO availability by supplying its principal NO-donor sources in the diet, typically L-arginine or vegetable-based nitrates, and now we can also add flaxseed to the list of NO-donor supplements.

3.3 BOTTOM LINE ... THE ENDOTHELIUM

It is important to understand the contribution to vascular physiology made by the discovery of the biological role of NO. But, it is largely left unsaid that this discovery simultaneously led to an even more important "discovery"—namely, the biological role of the *endothelium*, a single cell layer that lines the inside of blood vessels, lymphatic ducts, the heart (where it is termed the endocardium), the penis *cavernosae* (likewise in the clitoris) and other vascular structures. The word "discovery" is in quotes here because the cell structure of the endothelium was known, but it was thought to have no particular function other than a barrier "lining" the inner surface of arterial blood vessels in the vessel lumen.

NO is said to be a "signaling molecule" formed by the endothelium lining the arterial vascular system and the heart. Such molecules are released from the cells, sending the signal, crossing the gap between cells by diffusion and interacting with specific receptors in the cells that gave rise to them or other cells, triggering a response by activating a series of enzyme-controlled reactions that lead to changes in target cells.

While there may be a minor overlap in definition, *signal molecule* differs from *neurotransmitter molecule*. Signaling molecules transmit information between cells, some over short distances, while others transmit information over very long distances. Most neurotransmitters, on the other hand, are released at the end of a nerve fiber by the arrival of a nerve impulse and diffuse across the synapse or junction, causing the transfer of the impulse to another nerve fiber, a muscle fiber or some other structure.

3.3.1 THE STRUCTURE AND FUNCTION OF THE *ENDOTHELIUM*

Arterial blood vessels have three major structures: The innermost layer, the *tunica intima* (also called *tunica interna*), is simple squamous epithelium surrounded by a connective tissue basement membrane with elastic fibers. The middle layer, the *tunica media*, is primarily smooth muscle and is usually the thickest layer. It not only provides support for the vessel but also changes vessel diameter to regulate blood flow and blood pressure. The outermost layer, which attaches the vessel to the surrounding tissue, is the *tunica externa* or *tunica adventitia*. This layer is connective tissue with varying amounts of elastic and collagenous fibers. The connective tissue in this layer is quite dense where it is adjacent to the tunica media, but it changes to loose connective tissue near the periphery of the vessel.

In ordinary circumstances, the degree of constriction, or *tonus*, of arterial blood vessels and, consequently, blood flow and pressure, is determined by activity level in two control systems:

- The endothelium-independent system of action-hormones (adrenaline, nor-adrenalin, etc.) and diuresis, and
- The endothelium-dependent signal system based on the availability of NO, produced by the endothelium.

Figure 3.1 is an electron micrograph of a cross-section of a blood vessel: The red blood cells are shown in the *lumen* through which blood flows. The fluted accordion-like structure is the *endothelium* cell lining, surrounded by the blood vessel walls. The folds, or fluting, facilitate relaxation and thus enlargement of the vessel increasing blood flow.

It should be noted that the availability of L-arginine is never the only limiting factor in delivering NO. Endothelium dysfunction is another cause, and it was reported in a previous publication (4) that the limitations may also be due also to conditions that *unlink* or otherwise disable the eNOS enzyme (see the following discussion) that cleaves NO from L-arginine.

Many studies support the beneficial role of both omega-3 PUFAs and L-arginine in treatments of conditions that damage the endothelium and impair NO formation, including the following.

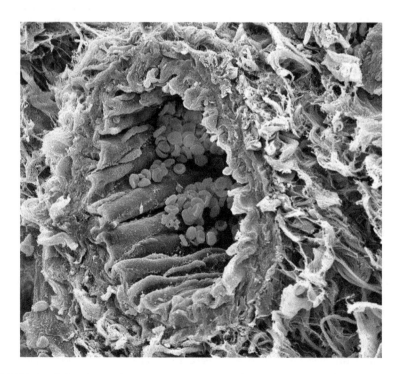

FIGURE 3.1 Colored scanning electron micrograph (SEM) of a sectioned artery containing red blood cells (erythrocytes). The fluting of the endothelium, the inner lining of the blood vessel, like that in an accordion, permits it to expand. [From Steve Gschmeissner. Science Photo Library. (3) With permission.]

A clinical study published in the journal *Atherosclerosis* in 2014 reported that "Omega-3 PUFAs improved endothelial function and arterial stiffness with a parallel anti-inflammatory effect in adults with metabolic syndrome." (47) And a clinical study published in the *International Journal of Cardiology* in 2002 reported, "Oral L-arginine improves endothelial dysfunction in patients with essential hypertension." (48)

A clinical study published in the *American Journal of Physiology. Heart and Circulatory Physiology* in 2018 titled "Flaxseed: Its Bioactive Components and Their Cardiovascular Benefits" reported that impaired vascular reactivity that accompanies atherosclerosis was also improved in both contraction and endothelium-dependent vessel relaxation in the presence of a flaxseed-supplemented diet. (49)

3.4 HOW DOES THE BODY FORM NO?

In the early 1900s, the Austrian pharmacologist Otto Loewi discovered a substance made by cells in the nervous system that he termed *"vagus material."* Some years later, Sir Henry Dale, with whom he later collaborated at the University of London, and with whom he shared the 1936 Nobel Prize in Medicine, named it "acetylcholine" (ACh). This was the beginning of neuropharmacology based on *neurotransmitter* chemical signals by which cells in the nervous system and the brain are now known to communicate.

ACh was found to relax arterial smooth muscles, and this seemed a promising road to lower blood pressure to treat hypertension. However, it did so unreliably and unpredictably. No one knew why. Then in 1980, Dr. Robert F. Furchgott, professor of pharmacology at Downstate Medical Center in Brooklyn, New York, published his findings in the journal *Nature* that ACh relaxation of arterial smooth muscle depended on the simultaneous presence of a mysterious substance formed by the endothelium. It was termed *"endothelium-derived relaxing factor"* (EDRF): ACh relaxed the vessels only when EDRF was also present. (5) The identity of EDRF was a mystery.

It did not take long to verify the finding, and in 1993, Dr. Salvador Moncada at Wellcome Research Labs, United Kingdom, who had previously first identified EDRF as the gas NO, detailed its role in health and disease in the *New England Journal of Medicine* (NEJM). (6)

In 1998, Dr. Furchgott and two colleagues, Louis J. Ignarro and Ferid Murad, were awarded the Nobel Prize in Medicine for the discovery of the biological role of NO in blood vessel relaxation. One of the three recipients, Dr. Louis J. Ignarro, later detailed how, in sexual arousal, ACh caused increased and sustained production of NO formed from the amino acid L-arginine by the endothelium lining the spongy chambers of the penis cavernosa(e). Following sexual stimulation, this causes them to relax (dilate), allowing increased blood inflow and thus erection. This discovery led to the development of Viagra®.

3.4.1 FOOTNOTE TO HISTORY

Why doesn't ACh reliably cause vasodilation in human blood circulation or in blood vessel strips in the laboratory? What Dr. Furchgott discovered in his strips of arterial blood vessels washed with ACh that did not relax is that on closer examination, it was found that "careless" laboratory preparation had damaged the endothelium, and it turns out that damaged endothelium impairs NO production.

The observation that damaged endothelium cannot produce NO in amounts sufficient to cause dilation and maintain adequate blood circulation is now the explanation for how we come by cardiovascular disorders such as hypertension, atherosclerosis, coronary heart disease, heart failure, kidney failure and the most common form of erectile dysfunction (ED), i.e., vasculogenic ED.

NO deficiency caused by damaged endothelium is at the core of most of the common health hazards, starting with hypertension, atherosclerosis and so on. And clearly, the damage to the endothelium is caused by a form equivalent to "careless" handling, our junk food diet poor in nutrients and antioxidants resulting often in *oxidative stress*.

3.5 REACTIVE OXYGEN SPECIES (ROS) AND OXIDATIVE STRESS—A MAJOR CAUSE OF ENDOTHELIUM DAMAGE

All the previously listed blood vessel damage conditions, and then some, are now said to be either due to or aggravated by oxidative stress. The principal damage is done to the endothelium. Oxidative stress results from sustained exposure to ROS that exceeds our antioxidant defense capability.

ROS are toxic compounds formed by oxygen free radicals, i.e., atoms, ions or molecules that have at least one unpaired electron in their structure, in combination with lipids, proteins or other substances. For instance, unpaired electrons reacting chemically with lipids cause lipid peroxidation, a damaging ROS.

The body ordinarily aims to neutralize or eliminate ROS to control their damaging effects. This ongoing battle that could ultimately deplete antioxidant defenses causes oxidative stress. Oxidative stress is the cost to the body of waging that battle. Oxidative stress damages the endothelium, reducing its ability to form NO by impairing endothelium function as surely as if it were mechanically damaged by "carelessly" mishandling in the laboratory.

It should be noted, however, that "carelessly" is not really accurate since no one had any idea then that the endothelium had any biological function, so why bother to spare it? It was thought then to be not much more than a sort of lining between the bloodstream and the blood vessel walls—a barrier, something like a bedsheet.

Flaxseed supplies antioxidant omega-3 PUFAs and L-arginine. In type 2 diabetes, ROS play a significant role in damaging blood vessel endothelium, thus fostering the development of conditions such a retinopathy. A study published in the *International Journal of Preventive Medicine*, in 2013, titled "The Effect of Omega-3 Supplements on Antioxidant Capacity in Patients with Type 2 Diabetes," concluded that omega-3 supplements can increase antioxidant capacity and that consumption of omega-3 supplements is recommended as primary prevention and secondary prevention of diabetes complications. (50)

Sickle cell disease entails endothelium activation and cell adhesion. (51) A report in the *Nutrition and Food Science International Journal* in 2019 titled "Antisickling and Antioxidant Properties of Omega-3 Fatty Acids EPA/DHA" concluded that omega-3 fatty acids EPA/DHA have antisickling, anti-hemolytic and antioxidant properties, reducing the number of crises in this disease. (52)

L-arginine is an antioxidant. The authors of a report titled "Arginine and Endothelial Function," published in the journal *Biomedicines* in 2020, contend that impaired endothelial NO availability in "perturbed vasculature" is likely due to diminished NO bioavailability or, indirectly, to increased ROS production that inactivates NO formation. They hold that in addition to counteracting oxidative stress, L-arginine supplementation represents an alternative potential therapeutic strategy in many cardiovascular disorders. (53)

There are a number of studies that report beneficial effects of flaxseed on endothelial function, but they are mostly experimental animal-model studies.

3.6 ENDOTHELIAL NO FROM L-ARGININE—NITRIC OXIDE SYNTHASE (eNOS)

The cells of the endothelium typically form NO from dietary L-arginine or nitrates with the help of synthase enzymes. There are three known (iso-)forms of the enzyme nitric oxide synthase (NOS): two are *constitutive* (cNOS) and the third is *inducible* (iNOS). The cNOS forms have two functions, one is brain constitutive, and the other is endothelial constitutive (eNOS). The third form is the inducible iNOS, which supplies the immune system cells with NO. Figure 3.2 illustrates NOS form and function.

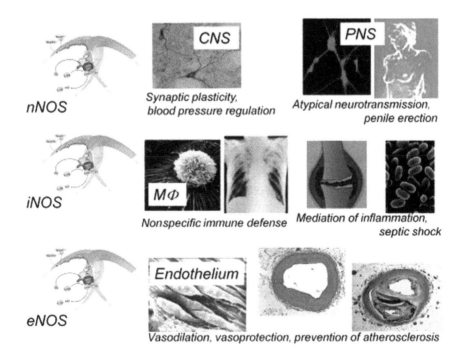

FIGURE 3.2 Important functions of the three known NOS isoforms. [Förstermann and Sessa. 2012. (7) *European Heart Journal*. With permission.]

In the top panel of Figure 3.2, neuronal NOS is shown to be expressed in specific neurons of the central nervous system involved in learning and memory formation. It also participates in the central control of blood pressure. In the peripheral nervous system, neuronal NOS-derived NO acts as an atypical neurotransmitter mediating relaxing components of gut peristalsis, and vasodilation.

In the middle panel of Figure 3.2, NOS expression can be induced by cytokines and other agents in almost any cell type. This had initially been shown for macrophages MΦ.

The MΦ-type of macrophage is an essential cellular first responder in the innate immune system, sensing, alerting, removing and destroying intracellular and extracellular pathogens. The induction of inducible NOS in MΦ is essential for the control of intracellular bacteria, such as *Mycobacterium tuberculosis* or the parasite *Leishmania*. However, inducible NOS is also up-regulated in various types of inflammatory diseases, and the NO generated by the enzyme mediates various symptoms of inflammation. Finally, inducible NOS-derived NO is the predominant mediator of vasodilation and blood pressure drop seen in septic shock.

The bottom panel of Figure 3.2 shows that endothelial NOS-derived NO is a physiological vasodilator but can also convey vasoprotection in several ways. NO released toward the vascular lumen is a potent inhibitor of platelet aggregation and adhesion to the vascular wall. Besides protection from thrombosis, this also prevents the release of platelet-derived growth factors that stimulate smooth muscle proliferation and its production of matrix molecules.

Endothelial NO also controls the expression of genes involved in atherogenesis. NO decreases the expression of chemoattractant protein MCP-1 and of a number of surface adhesion molecules, thereby preventing leucocyte adhesion to vascular endothelium and leucocyte migration into the vascular wall. This offers protection against early phases of atherogenesis. Also, the decreased endothelial permeability, the reduced influx of lipoproteins into the vascular wall and the inhibition of low-density lipoprotein oxidation may contribute to the anti-atherogenic properties of endothelial NOS-derived NO.

Finally, NO has been shown to inhibit DNA synthesis, mitogenesis and proliferation of vascular smooth muscle cells, as well as smooth muscle cell migration, thereby protecting against a later phase of atherogenesis. (7)

This description of the synthase enzymes clearly points to a key regulatory role for NO in virtually all body functions. But while brain and nervous system functions are of great interest, the focus of this book will be on cardiovascular, heart and kidney function, and by the way, eNO regulates blood vessel function in the cavernosa(e) of the penis and the clitoris in sexual arousal as well.

3.7 HOW ENDOTHELIUM-DERIVED NITRIC OXIDE (eNO) IS FORMED

Specifically, *endothelium*-derived NO forms in response to stimulation of the *endothelial* cells by cholinergic nerves. *Acetylcholine* causes the production of *inositol triphosphate* (IP3), a second messenger in many hormone signal transduction pathways. IP3 opens calcium channels in the endoplasmic membrane of the endothelial cells; the liberated calcium then activates NO synthase (eNOS) and causes the production of NO.

NO diffuses across the muscle cell membrane and binds to *guanylyl cyclase*. *Guanylyl cyclase* in turn catalyzes the synthesis of *cyclic guanosine monophosphate* (cGMP) from *guanosine triphosphate* (GTP). cGMP then activates a cGMP-dependent *protein kinase*, which stimulates the uptake of calcium by the endoplasmic reticulum of the smooth muscle cell. The reduced levels of cytoplasmic calcium cause the muscle cell to relax.

Vasodilation results from muscle cell relaxation, and, as is true of any signaling pathway, there must be a way to terminate the action of the signal: cGMP is converted into GMP by a specific *phosphodiesterase* (PDE). There are ten families of PDEs: PDE1–10. The major PDE in vascular smooth muscle is type 5. Viagra® (Sildenafil) is a specific inhibitor of PDE type 5. By blocking the breakdown of cGMP, Viagra acts to prolong the effects of cGMP, thus slowing the degradation of NO and so maintaining cavernosal blood inflow.

3.8 NO FORMED FROM CNglcs

Endothelium-derived nitric oxide (eNO) is a key signaling molecule in human cardiovascular physiology. It regulates blood circulation and the workload of the heart. But NO, otherwise derived, also plays an important role in plant physiology. There is now general agreement that NO is an important and almost universal signaling molecule in plants as well.

The role of NO in plants appears even more multifaceted than that in animals. Plant-borne NO seems involved in controlling cell differentiation and lignification, root and shoot development, flowering, growth and reorientation of pollen tubes, senescence and maturation, stomatal movement, plant-pathogen interactions and programmed cell death and many others. (8–12) There is little doubt that NO is an important second messenger. (13)

Flaxseeds, as do most plants to a lesser extent, hold CNglcs. Cyanide is formed following the hydrolysis of CNglcs that occurs during the crushing of the edible plant material (such as flaxseeds) either during consumption or during processing of the food crop. CNglcs can generate hydrocyanic acid (prussic acid, cyanide) when hydrolyzed by the enzyme beta-glucosidase into cyanohydrin. This is unstable and dissociates to hydrocyanic acid.

As previously noted, common CNglcs include amygdalin found in bitter almonds and peach kernels (both used in Chinese medicine), and prunasin in wild cherry bark (*Prunus serotina*). The small quantities of cyanide generated from this bark are said to be responsible for its antitussive properties, although this has not been confirmed in modern pharmacological experiments. In general, the effects of cyanide are dose related: in minute quantities, it stimulates respiration; in larger doses, it inhibits respiration; in larger doses yet, it is fatal.

Both amygdalin and prunasin yield benzaldehyde on hydrolysis, which accounts for the characteristic almond-like aroma of wild cherry bark. The CNglcs linustatin, neolinustatin and linamarin (in trace amounts) are found in flaxseeds (*Linum usitatissimum*).

Hydrolysis of the glycosides in the digestive tract or by the liver leads to a slow release of hydrocyanic acid that is readily detoxified by the body. In fact, amygdalin given orally to humans at 500 mg three times per day produced no toxic effects and only moderately raised blood cyanide levels. (14, 15)

3.9 THE BLOOD VESSELS OF THE BLOOD VESSELS (*VASA VASORUM*) ARE REGULATED BY NO

In considering diagnosis and treatment of blood vessel and heart disease, many clinical publications now focus on endothelial dysfunction. For instance, in 2014, the journal *Global Cardiology, Science, and Practice* published a report titled "Endothelial Dysfunction and Cardiovascular Disease." The term "endothelium" appeared 18 times in that article, and they tell us that the endothelium is a single vessel layer between the bloodstream and the vascular supply to other tissues. The endothelium is comprised of up to [a] trillion cells and it has the largest area in the body, covering 3 sq. meters and weighing in at about 1kg. It interacts with nearly every system in the body, and it is implicated in numerous disease including heart, neurologic, kidney, liver, blood vessels, skin and immunology-related disorders, but first and foremost is the hemostasis between thrombosis and anticoagulation. In addition, the endothelium regulates vascular tone by balancing vasoconstriction and vasodilation to provide adequate perfusion pressure to target organs. (2) Other functions include regulation of angiogenesis, wound healing, smooth muscle cell proliferation, fibrosis, and inflammation. The endothelium is adversely affected by cardiovascular risk factors such as tobacco use, obesity, age, hypertension, hyperlipidemia, physical inactivity, and poor dietary habits. It is positively affected by beneficial lifestyle habits such as increased physical activity, dietary habits which include anti-inflammatory and antioxidant foods, and some pharmaceutical agents such as L-arginine. (16)

The assertion that "the endothelium is a single vessel layer standing as the ultimate layer between blood and vascular supply to other tissues " is not actually accurate. If all goes well, the endothelium should not in fact come into contact with blood in the lumen because there is an additional structure, the glycocalyx, that separates the endothelium from blood in the vessel (see the following).

The authors of that paper (affiliated with the Mayo Clinic) curiously refer to L-arginine as a "pharmaceutical agent." It should be noted that exogenous L-arginine is not conventionally considered a pharmaceutical agent in the United States. Here, it is usually a "supplement." As will be shown later, its supplementation is repeatedly shown to significantly improve blood pressure and heart health. (17)

Arterial blood vessels and the endothelium, in particular, derive O_2 and nutrients and eliminate CO_2 and wastes only in small part by diffusion in and out of the blood vessel via the endothelium into and out of the bloodstream. The endothelium is additionally separated from the bloodstream by the glycocalyx, a carbohydrate-rich layer lining the vascular endothelium that forms a barrier to substance diffusion between the cells of the endothelium and the bloodstream in the vessel lumen. It is also subject to oxidative damage. More about that later.

3.9.1 STRUCTURE AND FUNCTION OF *VASA VASORUM*

Arterial blood vessel walls and the endothelium are supplied by their own set of blood vessels, the *vasa vasorum*, that draw blood from the bloodstream and deliver it to the vessel wall both inside and outside the walls.

The vasa vasorum is a network of small blood vessels that supply the walls of large blood vessels, such as elastic arteries (e.g., the aorta) and large veins (e.g., the venae cavae). There are two sets of these vessels, one set outside, the other inside. Figure 3.3 depicts a segment of normal (pig) coronary artery showing the origin and spatial distribution of vasa vasorum.

Vasa vasorum are dead-end structures. Unlike other aspects of blood circulation, there are no other means of return. Damaging atherogenic substances can enter blood vessel walls via the *vasa vasorum*. In fact, that is now thought to be the principal basis for atherosclerosis: attack from within. (19) The scenario goes something like this:

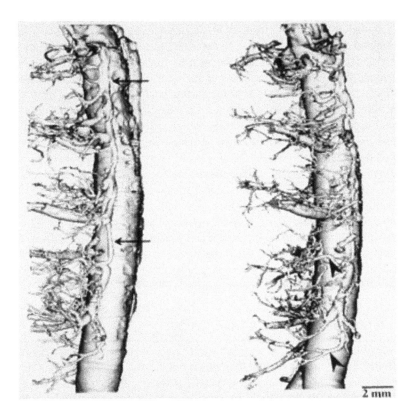

FIGURE 3.3 Micrographs showing voxel gradient shading of a normal coronary artery at different angles. Two anatomically different vasa types can be seen. First-order vasa vasorum (arrows) originate from branches of a coronary artery and run longitudinally to the main lumen. Second-order vasa vasorum (arrowheads) originate from first-order vasa and run circumferentially around the lumen, forming arch arterioles. Voxel size, 28 mm. [(18) *The Journal of Clinical Investigation*. With permission.]

Gradually, enlarging plaque deposits in the muscle wall distance the endothelium from the vasa vasorum and thus distances the endothelium from its source of O_2 while at the same time forcing it to encroach into the lumen. Thus metabolically jeopardized cells in the endothelium gradually lose their ability to form NO, and, ultimately, it may weaken and rupture due to shear stress on the inward bulge.

3.9.2 Vasa Vasorum Depends Exclusively on Endothelium-Derived (NO) Vasorelaxation

Both hypertension and atherosclerosis are known to damage the endothelium. In a study titled "On the Regulation of Tone in Vasa Vasorum" published in *Cardiovascular Research*, it was shown that vasa vasorum relaxation was solely endothelium-dependent—that is, NO-dependent—whereas the arterial vessel responded to both endothelium-dependent and the endothelium-independent relaxation signals (20) described next. In brief, the study also concluded that damage done by atherosclerosis to the endothelium intimately involves first changes in the vasa vasorum.

Writing in the journal *Medical Hypotheses* in 2009, researchers contend that known risk factors for atherosclerosis, such as high blood pressure and nicotine, reduce blood flow in the end branches of the vasa vasorum. Local impaired blood flow affects the cells of the endothelium causing local inflammation. This makes the endothelium permeable to large particles, such as various bacteria and low-density lipoproteins (LDL) and other fatty acids, which macrophages engulf transforming them into the *foam cells* that invade arterial blood vessel walls and begin the formation of plaque. (21)

These and many such reports underscore the dependence of arterial blood vessels on NO availability. While we understand that blood flow through a vessel depends on the ability of the endothelium of the vessel to form NO, it is equally clear that it is also dependent on the ability of the vasa vasorum that serves it to form NO.

NO unavailability in the vasa vasorum can be seen to begin a cascade of failures. This condition can be expected when the supply of the principal substrate for NO, L-arginine, is restricted due to a low protein diet (for reasons good or bad). These findings make a strong case for the importance of flaxseed as a NO-donor.

3.10 THE ENDOTHELIAL GLYCOCALYX

The endothelial glycocalyx is a carbohydrate-rich layer forming a lining covering the endothelium in the lumen and thus separating it from the bloodstream. It is connected to the endothelium through several "backbone" molecules, mainly proteins (proteoglycans), and glycoproteins, proteins forming a network in which soluble molecules, either plasma- or endothelium-derived, are incorporated. Figure 3.4 depicts the structure of the glycocalix.

Glycocalyx/eSL (endothelial surface layer) thickness is substantially greater than endothelial cell (eC) thickness, as demonstrated in a transmission electron micrograph of a goat coronary capillary (prepared using glycocalyx-sparing fixation techniques). Scale bar: 0.2 μm. Source: Yang and Schmidt. 2013. *Tissue Barriers*. (23) With permission.

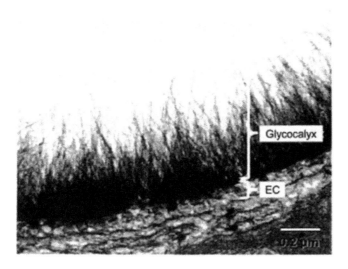

FIGURE 3.4 Structure of the endothelial surface layer showing the glycocalyx. [(18) *Journal of Clinical Investigation*. With permission.]

The endothelial glycocalyx is an intricate, self-assembling 3D mesh of various polysaccharides. A dynamic equilibrium exists between this layer of soluble components and the flowing blood continuously affecting composition and thickness of the glycocalyx. Several of its specific properties are worth mentioning.

The endothelial glycocalyx is the endothelial gatekeeper. Located in the lumen between the bloodstream and the endothelium, it is an important determinant of vascular permeability. It can limit access of certain molecules to the endothelial cell membrane, and it has been shown that enzymatic (partial) removal and subsequent loss of permeability barrier function of the glycocalyx leads to myocardial edema. (24)

The presence of a relatively thick endothelial glycocalyx *in vivo* has great consequences for the deformation of blood vessels and blood flow characteristics (rheology), especially in the microvasculature. In this part of the circulation, local blood viscosity and hematocrit (density of red blood cells in the area) appear to be modulated by the glycocalyx.

Besides its capacity to restrict molecules from reaching the endothelium, the glycocalyx also influences blood cell—vessel wall interactions. It repulses red blood cells from the endothelium. In the microcirculation, a red blood cell exclusion zone flanking the endothelium can be observed *in vivo*, which is decreased upon breakdown of the glycocalyx. Similarly, platelets are not often observed interacting with the endothelium in control conditions, whereas partial glycocalyx removal is accompanied by an increase in platelet-vessel wall interactions, which are dangerous because they favor clot formation.

Cells defective of glycosylation, having a thinner glycocalyx, showed increased attachment of neutrophils. Hence, in normal conditions, the soluble components of the glycocalyx seem to shield adhesion molecules, thereby preventing interaction. Stimuli that degrade the glycocalyx or induce a more open mesh, such as enzymes, cytokines or ischemia and reperfusion, appear to uncover the adhesion molecules, which, in turn, allows blood cells to interact with the endothelium, which, again, is bad because it favors clot formation. (22)

The endothelial glycocalyx is a mechanotransducer. Endothelial cells exposed to shear stress produce NO, an important determinant of vascular tone. Shear stress is caused by the flow of fluid across a surface, and its value is directly proportional to the velocity of the surrounding fluid.

Recently, the glycocalyx has been added to the list of possible candidates responsible for the translation of biomechanical forces into biochemical signals. (5) It appears that shear stress is transmitted to other regions of the endothelial cell as well, such as intercellular junctions and basal adhesion plaques, which are responsible for additional shear sensing, even in the absence of a glycocalyx. (26)

The endothelial glycocalyx also controls the microenvironment. Docking of plasma-derived molecules can influence the local environment in several ways: Binding of receptors or enzymes and their ligands to the endothelial glycocalyx causes a localized rise in the concentration of these substances. This enables proper signaling or enzymatic modification.

Several important anticoagulant mediators such as antithrombin III, heparin cofactor II, thrombomodulin and tissue factor pathway inhibitor can bind to the glycocalyx making it vasculoprotective. Antithrombin III is a strong inhibitor of procoagulant enzymes like thrombin and activated factors X and IX (FXa and FIXa). (27) All anticoagulant molecules present in the glycocalyx contribute to the thromboresistant nature of healthy endothelium. (28) The endothelial glycocalyx also modulates inflammatory responses by binding cytokines and attenuating binding of cytokines to cell surface receptors.

Another aspect of the vasculoprotective role of the endothelial glycocalyx is that it supports antioxidant activity by binding quenchers of oxygen radicals, such as extracellular superoxide dismutase (SOD). (29) These enzymes help to reduce the oxidative stress and keep up NO bioavailability, thus, preventing the endothelium from becoming dysfunctional.

3.10.1 The Glycocalyx Regulates eNO Formation

It is hard to imagine that the glycocalyx, this ultrathin mushy layer, could have so many and such varied endothelium-protective activities. As noted earlier, one of these is mechanical, i.e., it protects the endothelium from the fluid shear stress caused by blood flowing through the lumen. As noted previously, degradation of the glycocalyx promotes atherogenesis and exposes the endothelium to shear stress incurring the risk of rupture. This finding links diabetes, for instance, to "coronary" heart attack, an otherwise unclear connection. And, parenthetically, the glycocalyx gradually becomes dysfunctional as the vasculature ages. That dysfunction contributes to impairment of endothelial NO formation. (30)

Investigators reporting in the *Biophysical Journal* concluded that the glycocalyx is a significant mediator of NO production in endothelial cells; degradation of the endothelial glycocalyx layer drastically reduces endothelial cells production of NO in response to fluid shear stress. (31) And in the journal *PLoS One*, investigators reported a study concluding that endothelial surface glycocalyx (ibid.) participates in endothelial cell mechanosensing and transduction through its heparan sulfate to activate eNOS. (25, 32)

3.11 THE ENDOTHELIAL GLYCOCALYX IN HEALTH AND DISEASE

In healthy vessels, the endothelial glycocalyx determines vascular permeability, attenuates blood cell–vessel wall interactions, mediates shear stress sensing, enables balanced signaling and fulfills a vasculoprotective role. But when it is disrupted or modified, these properties are lost, as has been shown through direct targeting of the glycocalyx in experimental settings. In the last few years, evidence has been emerging that (damage to) the glycocalyx plays a pivotal role in several vascular pathologies.

3.11.1 Diabetes

One of the hallmarks of diabetes is insulin insufficiency or resistance, and subsequent hyperglycemia, impairing the protective capacity of the vessel wall and resulting in enhanced endothelial permeability and impaired NO synthase function. (33) However, a common pathway leading to these vascular dysfunctions has not been identified.

It was recently shown that the systemic glycocalyx volume of healthy volunteers, as assessed by comparing the intravascular distribution volume of a glycocalyx-permeable and a glycocalyx-impermeable tracer, declined to one-half the volume six hours after induction of acute hyperglycemia. (34) Using the same methodology, the systemic glycocalyx volume in Type 1 diabetes patients was found to be about half of that of healthy controls; it was further reduced in those with microalbuminuria. (35)

In the same study, plasma levels of hyaluronan and hyaluronidase were found to be elevated in patients with diabetes, reflecting increased synthesis and shedding of hyaluronan under hyperglycemic conditions.

> *Hyaluronan (hyaluronic acid) is a high-molecular-mass polysaccharide found in the extracellular matrix, especially of soft connective tissues. It is synthesized in the plasma membrane of fibroblasts and other cells by the addition of sugars to the reducing end of the polymer, whereas the nonreducing end protrudes into the pericellular space. The polysaccharide is catabolized locally or carried by lymph to lymph nodes or the general circulation from where it is cleared by the endothelial cells of the liver sinusoids. Hyaluronan has been assigned various physiological functions in the intercellular matrix, e.g., in water and plasma protein homeostasis.*

Analysis of serum hyaluronan is promising in the diagnosis of liver disease and various inflammatory conditions, e.g., rheumatoid arthritis. Interstitial edema caused by accumulation of hyaluronan may cause dysfunction in various organs. (36)

Both studies showed that acute and long-standing hyperglycemia is associated with profound reduction of glycocalyx volume. It is tempting to speculate that this damage to the glycocalyx contributes to endothelial dysfunction in hyperglycemic conditions, which can be measured in nondiabetic individuals as well. In fact, postprandial hyperglycemia, induced by oral glucose loading, attenuates endothelial function as measured by decreased flow-mediated dilation (FMD) in healthy individuals without diabetes. (37)

> *FMD refers to dilation of an artery when blood flow increases in that artery. The primary mechanism of FMD is the release of NO by endothelial cells.*

3.11.2 Atherosclerosis

Atherosclerosis is a large artery disease marked by disturbed blood flow profiles. There is evidence that the endothelial glycocalyx is involved in atherogenesis. One study reported that administration of clinically relevant doses of oxidized LDL leads to a disruption of the glycocalyx in hamster cremaster muscle microcirculation and evokes local platelet adhesion. However, co-infusion with the antioxidant enzymes SOD and catalase, enzymes catalyzing the dismutation of superoxide anion and the decomposition of hydrogen peroxide abolished this effect, implicating a role for oxygen-derived free radicals in the genesis of atherosclerosis. (38)

Apparently, loss of glycocalyx results in loss of endogenous protective enzymes, such as extracellular SOD, and that increases the oxidative stress on endothelial cells. This was further illustrated in a recent study showing a reduction in glycocalyx dimensions after a high-fat diet. (39)

In another study, an inverse relation between glycocalyx thickness and blood vessel intima-media ratio was found, reflecting a reduction of vasculoprotective capacity of the endothelial glycocalyx at sites with higher atherogenic risk. (40) These studies suggest the rather novel notion that the endothelial glycocalyx is involved in the initiation and progression of the atherosclerotic process.

3.11.3 Hypertension

It is reasonably well established that a high-salt diet is one of the major risk factors in the development and maintenance of hypertension. Numerous experimental and observational studies have confirmed the association of sodium intake with blood pressure levels. The effects of a high-salt diet are related to the function of the renin-angiotensin system, which is normally suppressed by a high-salt diet. Endothelial dysfunction probably plays an important role in the influence of high sodium intake on blood pressure.

The renin-angiotensin-aldosterone system (RAAS) is a critical regulator of blood volume and systemic vascular resistance. While the baroreceptor reflex responds in a short-term manner to decreased arterial pressure, the RAAS is responsible for more chronic alterations. It is composed of three major compounds: renin, angiotensin II and aldosterone. These three act to elevate arterial pressure in response to decreased renal blood pressure, decreased salt delivery to the distal convoluted tubule and/or beta-adrenergic agonism. Through these mechanisms, the body can elevate the blood pressure in a prolonged manner.

This is the common wisdom underlying management of hypertension. But recent studies of the glycocalyx unearthed another source of cardiovascular damage attributable to excessive salt intake:

According to a report in the journal *F1000 Reports Biology*, salt entering the vascular bed after a salty meal is bound to the endothelial glycocalyx. This barrier protects the endothelium against salt overload. But a degraded glycocalyx increases the salt permeability of the vascular system and the amount of salt being deposited in the body, which affects organ function. (41)

These findings may shed some light on why salt loading results in a decrease in NO production in both salt-sensitive and salt-resistant normotensive individuals, which is independent of changes in blood pressure. (42)

In connection with management of chronic hypertension, it should be noted that increasing salt concentration by as little as 4 mM (about one four hundredths of a teaspoon) immediately induces damage to glycocalyx leading to chronic Na^+ and Ca^{2+} overload and vascular smooth muscle cells hypertrophy. (43)

3.11.4 KIDNEY FUNCTION

NO has a key role in kidney function. It regulates renal haemodynamics, maintains perfusion of the middle (medullary) part of the kidney, mediates pressure-natriuresis (i.e., excretion of salt), inhibits tubular sodium reabsorption and modulates renal sympathetic neural activity. Its principal effect is to promote natriuresis and diuresis. Deficient renal NO synthesis is implicated in the pathogenesis of hypertension. All three isoforms of nitric oxide synthase (NOS)—namely, neuronal NOS (nNOS or NOS1), inducible NOS (iNOS or NOS2) and endothelial NOS (eNOS or NOS3)—are reported to contribute to NO synthesis in the kidney. (44)

Finally, total NO production was found to be decreased in renal disease, likely due to impaired endothelial and renal NO production. (45)

Numerous clinical studies support supplementation of omega-3 fatty acids and L-arginine where deficient bioavailability of NO seems to be the principal culprit. Sometimes these studies cite flaxseed, *per se*, as the dependent variable. At other times, it is either omega-3 or L-arginine. There is a more detailed look at flaxseed constituents in common cardiovascular disorders in subsequent chapters.

3.12 SUMMARY

NO is a signal molecule ordinarily derived in the body from the amino acid L-arginine in common staple foods containing proteins and nitrates. And it is also available to body functions from both L-arginine and CNglcs (e.g. in flaxseed). NO is both formed by the vascular endothelium and acts on it to regulate blood flow. The vascular endothelium, in turn, largely depends for its blood supply on the *vasa vasorum*, which also both forms NO and depends on it for its vascular control activities.

The luminal surface of the endothelium is lined by the *glycocalyx*, which modulates endothelium NO formation and supplies antioxidant protection as well. A number of common health hazards are now linked to the degradation of the glycocalyx, which results in endothelium function impairment and due to, and consequently jeopardizing, production of endothelial NO. These hazards typically encompass the panoply of cardiovascular diseases involving blood vessels, heart and kidney dysfunctions and metabolic disorders, including type 2 diabetes.

Clinical trials have shown that flaxseed, *per se* omega-3 fatty acids and L-arginine, are antioxidants and, as such, supplementation has been recommended in support of endothelial NO synthesis commonly jeopardized by ROS in cardiovascular disorders.

3.13 REFERENCES

1. Taddei S, Virdis A, Ghiadoni L, Salvetti G, Bernini G, Magagna A, and A Salvetti. 2001. Age-related reduction of NO availability and oxidative stress in humans. *Hypertension*, 38: 274–279. DOI:10.1161/01.hyp.38.2.274.
2. https://slideplayer.com/slide/4562121/; accessed 1/21/20.
3. www.sciencephoto.com/media/303611/view/artery-sem.
4. Fried R, and RM Carlton. 2018. *Type 2 diabetes: Cardiovascular and related complications and evidence-based complementary treatments*. Boca Raton: CRC Press/Taylor & Francis.
5. Furchgott RF, and JV Zawadzki. 1980. The obligatory role of endothelial cells in the relaxation of arterial smooth muscle by acetylcholine. *Nature*, Nov; 288(5789): 373–376. DOI:10.1038/288373a0.
6. Moncada S, and EA Higgs, eds. 1990. *Nitric oxide from L-arginine: A bioregulatory system*. Amsterdam: Elsevier Science Publishers.
7. Förstermann U, and WC Sessa. 2012. Nitric oxide synthases: Regulation and function. *European Heart Journal*, Apr; 33(7): 829–837. DOI:10.1093/eurheartj/ehr304.
8. Becker WM, Kleinsmith, LJ, Hardin J, and GP Bertoni. 2008. *The world of the cell*, 7th ed. Copyright: Pearson Education Inc. email bestave@mun.ca. www.mun.ca/biology/desmid/brian/BIOL2060/BIOL2060-14/CB14old.html.
9. Lamattina L, García-Mata C, Graziano M, and G Pagnussat. 2003. Nitric oxide: The versatility of an extensive signal molecule. *Annual Review of Plant Biology*, 54: 109–136. DOI:10.1146/annurev.arplant.54.031902.134752.
10. Neill SJ, Desikan R, and JT Hancock. 2003. Nitric oxide signalling in plants. *New Phytologist*, 159: 11–35. DOI:10.1046/j.1469-8137.2003.00804.x.
11. Romero-Puertas MC, Perazzolli M, Zago ED, and M Delledonne. 2004. Nitric oxide signalling functions in plant-pathogen interactions. *Cellular Microbiology*, Sept; 6: 795–803. DOI:10.1111/j.1462-5822.2004.00428.x.
12. Wendehenne D, Durner J, and DF Klessig. 2004. Nitric oxide: A new player in plant signalling and defence responses. *Current Opinion in Plant Biology*, Aug; 7: 449–455. DOI:10.1016/j.pbi.2004.04.002.
13. Planchet E, and WM Kaiser. 2006. Nitric oxide production in plants. Facts and fictions. *Plant Signaling and Behaior*, Mar–Apr; 1(2): 46–51. DOI:10.4161/psb.1.2.2435.
14. Moertel CG, Ames MM, Kovach JS, Moyer TP, Rubin JR, and JH Tinker. 1981. A pharmacologic and toxicological study of amygdalin. *JAMA*, Feb; 245(6): 591–594. PMID: 7005480.

15. Bone K, and S Mills, eds. 2013. Cyanogenic glycoside. In: *Principles and practice of phytotherapy. Modern herbal medicine*, 2nd ed. Edinburgh: Churchill Livingstone, pp. 17–82. DOI:10.1016/B978-0-443-06992-5.00002-5.
16. Widmer RJ, and A Lerman. 2014. Endothelial dysfunction and cardiovascular disease. *Global Cardiology, Science, and Practice*, 2014(3): 291–308. DOI:10.5339/gcsp.2014.43.
17. Arginine: Heart benefits and side effects. www.webmd.com/heart/arginine-heart-benefits-and-side-effects#1; accessed 1/21/20.
18. Kwon HK, Sangiorgi G, Ritman EL, McKenna C, Holmes DR Jr, Schwartz RS, and A Lerman. 1998. Enhanced coronary vasa vasorum neovascularization in experimental hypercholesterolemia. *The Journal of Clinical Investigation*, Apr; 101(8): 1551–1556. www.sciencedirect.comscience/article/pii/S0735109798004823; accessed 1/21/20.
19. Sedding DG, Boyle EC, Demandt JAF, Sluimer JC, Dutzmann J, Haverich A, and J Bauersachs. 2018. Vasa vasorum angiogenesis: Key player in the initiation and progression of atherosclerosis and potential target for the treatment of cardiovascular disease. *Frontiers in Immunology*, Apr 17; 9: 706. DOI:10.3389/fimmu.2018.00706.
20. Scotland R, Vallance P, and A Ahluwalia. 1999. On the regulation of tone in vasa vasorum. *Cardiovascular Research*, Jan; 41(1): 237–245. DOI:10.1016/S0008-6363(98)00223-5.
21. Järvilehto M, and P Tuohimaa. 2009. Vasa vasorum hypoxia: Initiation of atherosclerosis. *Medical Hypotheses*, Jul; 73(1): 40–41. DOI:10.1016/j.mehy.2008.11.046.
22. Schmidt EP, Yang Y, Janssen WJ, Gandjeva A, Perez MJ, Barthel L, Zemans RL, Bowman JC, Koyanagi DE, Yunt ZX, Smith LP, Cheng SS, Overdier KH, Thompson KR, Geraci MW, Douglas IS, Pearse DB, and RM Tuder. 2012. The pulmonary endothelial glycocalyx regulates neutrophil adhesion and lung injury during experimental sepsis. *Nature Medicine*, Aug; 18(8): 1217–1223. DOI:10.1038/nm.2843.
23. Yang Y, and EP Schmidt. 2013. The endothelial glycocalyx: An important regulator of the pulmonary vascular barrier. *Tissue Barriers*, Jan 1; 1(1). e23494. DOI:10.4161/tisb.23494. www.ncbi.nlm.nih.gov/pubmed/24073386.
24. van den Berg BM, Vink H, and JAE Spaan. 2003. The endothelial glycocalyx protects against myocardial edema. *Circulation Research*, Mar; 92: 592–594. DOI:10.1161/01.RES.0000065917.53950.75.
25. Florian JA, Kosky JR, Ainslie K, Pang Z, Dull RO, and JM Tarbell. 2003. Heparan sulfate proteoglycan is a mechanosensor on endothelial cells. *Circulation Research*, Nov 14; 93(10): e136–142. DOI:10.1161/01.RES.0000101744.47866.D5.
26. Tarbell JM, and MY Pahakis. 2006. Mechanotransduction and the glycocalyx. *Journal of Internal Medicine*, Apr; 259(4): 339–350. DOI:10.1111/j.1365-2796.2006.01620.x.
27. Quinsey NS, Greedy AL, Bottomley SP, Whisstock JC, and RN Pike. 2004. Antithrombin: In control of coagulation. *International Journal of Biochemistry and Cell Biology*, Mar; 36(3): 386–339. DOI:10.1016/s1357-2725(03)00244-9.
28. Egbrink MG, Van Gestel MA, Broeders MA, Tangelder GJ, Heemskerk JM, Reneman RS, and DW Slaaf. 2005. Regulation of microvascular thromboembolism in vivo. *Microcirculation*, Apr–May; 12(3): 287–300. DOI:10.1080/10739680590925628.
29. Li Q, Bolli R, Qiu Y, Tang XL, Murphree SS, and BA French. 1998. Gene therapy with extracellular superoxide dismutase attenuates myocardial stunning in conscious rabbits. *Circulation*, Oct 6; 98(14): 1438–1448. DOI:10.1161/01.cir.98.14.1438.
30. Machin DR, Nguyen D, Colton Bramwell RC, Lesniewski LA, and AJ Donato. 2019. Dietary glycocalyx precursor supplementation ameliorates age-related vascular dysfunction. *FASEB*, 33(1): 828.1. DOI:10.1096/fasebj.2019.33.1_supplement.828.1.
31. Bartosch AMW, Mathews R, and JM Tarbell. 2017. Endothelial glycocalyx-mediated nitric oxide production in response to selective AFM pulling. *Biophysics Journal*, Jul 11; 113(1): 101–108. DOI:10.1016/j.bpj.2017.05.033.

32. Yen W, Cai B, Yang J, Zhang L, Zeng M, Tarbell JM, and BM Fu. 2015. Endothelial surface glycocalyx can regulate flow-induced nitric oxide production in microvessels in vivo. *PLoS ONE*, Jan 9; 10(1): e0117133. DOI:10.1371/journal.pone.0117133.
33. Du XL, Edelstein D, Dimmeler S, Ju Q, Sui C, and Brownlee M. 2001. Hyperglycemia inhibits endothelial nitric oxide synthase activity by posttranslational modification at the Akt site. *Journal of Clinical Investigation*, Nov; 108(9): 1341–1348. DOI:10.1172/JCI11235.
34. Nieuwdorp M, van Haeften TW, Gouverneur MC, Mooij HL, van Lieshout MH, Levi M, Meijers JC, Holleman F, Hoekstra JB, Vink H, Kastelein JJ, and ES Stroes. 2006. Loss of endothelial glycocalyx during acute hyperglycemia coincides with endothelial dysfunction and coagulation activation in vivo. *Diabetes*, Feb; 55(2): 480–486. DOI:10.2337/diabetes.55.02.06.db05-1103.
35. Nieuwdorp M, Mooij HL, Kroon J, Atasever B, Spaan JA, Ince C, Holleman F, Diamant M, Heine RJ, Hoekstra JB, Kastelein JJ, Stroes ES, and H Vink. 2005. Endothelial glycocalyx damage coincides with microalbuminuria in type 1 diabetes. *Diabetes*, Apr; 55(4): 1127–1132. DOI:10.2337/diabetes.55.04.06.db05-1619.
36. Laurent TC, and JR Fraser. 1992. Hyaluronan. *The FASEB Journal*, Apr; 6(7): 2397–2404. PMID: 1563592.
37. Title LM, Cummings PM, Giddens K, and BA Nassar. 2000. Oral glucose loading acutely attenuates endothelium-dependent vasodilation in healthy adults without diabetes: An effect prevented by vitamins C and E. *Journal of the American College of Cardiology*, Dec; 36(7): 2185–2191. DOI:10.1016/s0735-1097(00)00980-3.
38. Vink H, Constantinescu AA, and JA Spaan. 2000. Oxidized lipoproteins degrade the endothelial surface layer: Implications for platelet-endothelial cell adhesion. *Circulation*, Apr 4; 101(13): 1500–1502. DOI:10.1161/01.cir.101.13.1500.
39. van den Berg BM, Spaan JA, Rolf TM, and H Vink. 2006. Atherogenic region and diet diminish glycocalyx dimension and increase intima-to-media ratios at murine carotid artery bifurcation. *American Journal of Physiology, Heart and Circulation Physiology*, Feb; 290(2): H915–920. DOI:10.1152/ajpheart.00051.2005.
40. Nieuwdorp M, Meuwese MC, Vink H, Hoekstra JBL, Kastelein JJP, and ES Stroes. 2005. The endothelial glycocalyx: A potential arrier between health and vascular disease. *Current Opinion in Lipidology*, Oct; 16(5): 507–511. DOI:10.1097/01.mol.0000181325.08926.9c.
41. Kusche-Vihrog K, and H Oberleithner. 2012. An emerging concept of vascular salt sensitivity. *F1000 Reports Biology*, 4: 20. DOI:10.3410/B4-20.
42. Dishy V, Sofowora GG, Imamura H, Nishimi Y, Xie H-G, Wood AJ, and CM Stein. 2003. Nitric oxide production decreases after salt loading but is not related to blood pressure changes or nitric oxide-mediated vascular responses. *Journal of Hypertension*, Jan; 21(1): 153–157. DOI:10.1097/00004872-200301000-00025.
43. Bkaily G, Simon Y, Menkovic I, Bkaily C, and D Jacques. 2018. High salt-induced hypertrophy of human vascular smooth muscle cells associated with a decrease in glycocalyx. *Journal of Molecular and Cell Cardiology*, Dec; 125: 1–5. DOI:10.1016/j.yjmcc.2018.10.006.
44. Mount PF, and DA Power. 2006. Nitric oxide in the kidney: Functions and regulation of synthesis. *Acta Physiologica (Oxf)*, Aug; 187(4): 4334–4346. DOI:10.1111/j.1748-1716.2006.01582.x.
45. Baylis C. 2008. Nitric oxide deficiency in chronic kidney disease. *American Journal of Physiology—Renal Physiology*, Jan 1; 294(1): F1–F9. DOI:10.1152/ajprenal.00424.2007.
46. Cohn JN, McInnes GT, and AM Shepherd. 2011. Direct-acting vasodilators. *Clinical Hypertension (Greenwich)*, Sep; 13(9): 690–692. DOI:10.1111/j.1751-7176.2011.00507.x.

47. Tousoulis D, Plastiras A, Siasos G, Miliou A, Paraskevopoulos T, and C Stefanadis. 2014. Omega-3 PUFAs improved endothelial function and arterial stiffness with a parallel anti-inflammatory effect in adults with metabolic syndrome. *Atherosclerosis*, Jan 1; 232(1): 10–16. DOI:10.1016/j.atherosclerosis.2013.10.014.
48. Lekakis JP, Papathanassiou S, Papaioannou TG, Papamichael CM, Zakopoulos N, Kotsis V, Dagre AG, Stamatelopoulos K, Protogerou A, and SF Stamatelopoulos. 2002. Oral L-arginine improves endothelial dysfunction in patients with essential hypertension. *International Journal of Cardiology*, Dec; 86(2–3): 317–323. DOI:10.1016/s0167-5273(02)00413-8.
49. Parikh M, Netticada T, and GN Pierce. 2018. Flaxseed: Its bioactive components and their cardiovascular benefits. *American Journal of Physiology. Heart and Circulatory Physiology*, 314: H146–H159. DOI:10.1152/ajpheart.00400.2017.
50. Hajianfar H, Paknahad Z, and A Bahonar. 2013. The effect of omega-3supplements on antioxidant capacity in patients with Type 2 diabetes. *International Journal of Preventive Medicine*, May; 4(Suppl 2): S234–S238. PMCID: PMC3678224.
51. Kaul DK, Finnegan E, and GA Barabino. 2009. Sickle red cell—endothelium interaction. *Microcirculation*, Jan; 16(1): 97–111. DOI:10.1080/10739680802279394.
52. Kotue TC, Djote WNB, Marlyne M, Pieme AC, Kansci G, and E Fokou. 2019. Antisickling and antioxidant properties of omega-3 fatty acids EPA/DHA. *Nutrition and Food Science International Journal*, 9(1): 555752. DOI:10.19080/NFSIJ.2019.09.555752.
53. Gambardella J, Khondkar W, Morelli MB, Xujun Wang X, Santulli G, and V Trimarco. 2020. Arginine and endothelial function. *Biomedicines*, Aug; 8(8): 277. DOI:10.3390/biomedicines8080277.

4 The Role of Flaxseed Micronutrients and Nitric Oxide (NO) in Blood Vessel and Heart Function

It is ambition enough to be employed as an under-labourer in clearing the ground a little, and removing some of the rubbish which lies in the way to knowledge.

—John Locke (1689)

4.1 INTRODUCTION

The first three chapters of this book detailed the panoply of health-giving microconstituents in flaxseed and flax oil—many as antioxidants and others as a source of nitric oxide (NO), the latter derived from both L-arginine and cyanogenic glycosides (CNglcs). In general, flaxseed improves cardiovascular function:

A study published in the *American Journal of Physiology—Heart and Circulation Physiology* reports that a number of preclinical and clinical studies have shown the beneficial cardiovascular effects of dietary supplementation with flaxseed. They include

- Antihypertensive action
- Anti-atherogenic effects
- Cholesterol lowering
- Anti-inflammatory action
- Inhibition of arrhythmias

The investigators generally attribute these beneficial effects to enrichment with the omega-3 fatty acid, alpha-linolenic acid and the antioxidant lignin, secoisolariciresinol diglucoside (SDG), as well as its high fiber content. In addition, flaxseed holds other potential bioactive compounds, such as proteins, cyclolinopeptides, and CNglcs, which have been shown to produce biological effects. These compounds could also be responsible for the beneficial cardiovascular effects of flaxseed. (1)

The benefits of flaxseed supplementation derive in large part from increased endothelial NO (eNO) availability. But evidence-based reports of the benefits of flaxseed supplementation do not invariably identify these active constituents. More often, they focus on antioxidant capacity. This will be quite evident in studies cited throughout this book.

Maintaining viable eNO formation and availability in the cardiovascular system is absolutely essential, and an "amino acid deprivation diet," indicated in certain medical disorders can, under certain circumstances, results in NO insufficiency. An important example of an intentional amino acid deprivation diet is restricting dietary intake of amino acids. Amino acid restriction plays a key role in cancer interventions, including arginine starvation, glycine restriction, serine starvation, leucine deprivation glutamine blockade, asparagine and methionine restriction. (43) The consequences of such insufficiency to the viability of blood vessels and the heart cannot be overstated. Therefore, to head off NO insufficiency, both CNglcs and L-arginine from flaxseed supplementation are proposed as beneficial NO-donors.

This chapter first details the physiological components of blood circulation and its assessment critical to understanding how NO is the key to heart and blood vessel function. Then we will look at clinical reports of the benefits to eNO formation of supplementing flaxseed or its constituents, omega-3 fatty acids or L-arginine.

4.2 WHAT PROPELS BLOOD THROUGH THE CIRCULATORY SYSTEM?

On the face of it, the question "what propels blood through the circulatory system" must seem naïve. After all, it is well-known that it is the pumping action of the heart that sees to that. That's what Wm Harvey said in the mid-1600s. But in fact, not exactly.

4.2.1 Systole

The normal heart (Figure 4.1 is a "cutaway" illustration) has two upper and two lower chambers. The upper chambers, the right and left atria, receive incoming blood, shown in blue. Blue typically indicates that there is less than normal oxygen (O_2) content, whereas red indicates properly oxygenated blood. In fact, the veins in the wrist appear blue because veins usually carry less oxygenated blood than arteries.

The lower chambers, the more muscular right and left ventricles, pump blood out of the heart. The heart valves, which keep blood flowing in the right direction, are gates at the entrance to the chambers, preventing blood from flowing back when the ventricle chambers contract.

The action of the left ventricle (shown on the right in Figure 4.1) is of great concern because it can malfunction for various reasons thus seriously affecting blood circulation. One of those malfunctions is *heart failure*.

The adequacy of the pumping action of the heart is determined by what is known as the "ejection fraction"—that is, the amount—percentage actually—of blood that is pumped out (or ejected) by each contraction of the ventricle as a bolus into the aorta and thus into the bloodstream. The left ventricle does not eject all the blood it contains with each contraction and so the efficiency of the heart is determined by the percentage of the blood it contains that is actually "ejected" into the blood

The Role of Flaxseed Micronutrients in Blood Vessel and Heart Function

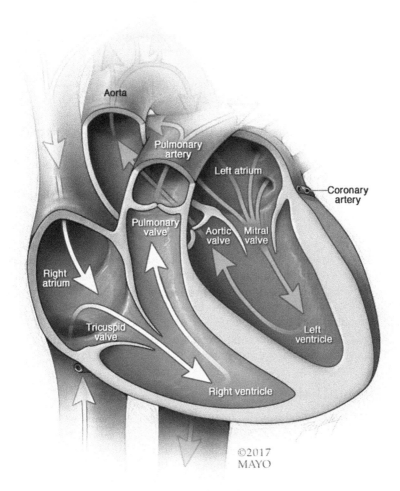

FIGURE 4.1 Chambers and valves of the heart. (From mayoclinic.org. With permission.)

circulation with each beat. A normal heart ejection fraction may be between 50% and 70%. Ejection fraction under 40% may be evidence of "heart failure."

Just as blood vessels have an endothelial lining that participates in the function of the vessel, the heart has a parallel inner surface lining, the *endocardium*. The *endocardium* consists of a layer of endothelial cells and an underlying layer of connective tissue. Therefore, the action of the heart, just like that of arterial blood vessels, is regulated not only by action-hormones but to a great extent by the activity of NO. And, just like blood vessels, its function is jeopardized by anything that affects the viability of endothelial cells and eNO formation. Reactive oxygen species (ROS) come to mind. (2, 3)

The adequacy of the pumping action of the heart also depends on the synchrony of the sequence of the chamber contractions. One study showed that one form of asynchrony (arrhythmia), the well-known and not so uncommon atrial fibrillation, disrupts the formation of NO by the endocardium. Apparently, atrial fibrillation reduces the ability of the endocardium to form NO as needed, and this can also lead to stroke. (4)

Blood flowing to the heart proper is delivered by the two-branch (right and left) coronary arteries encircling the surface of the heart.

When the heart contracts, i.e. systole, the aortic valve opens as it ejects a portion of the contents of the left ventricle into the aorta. Then the valve closes. Understanding what happens next is the key to understanding why NO is crucial to blood circulation. But exactly how dependent is heart function on NO availability?

According to a report in *Science Daily* (May 14, 2018), "Heart disease severity may depend on nitric oxide levels: Study finds nitric oxide may also determine drug efficacy." (5) The report informs us that not only is NO deficiency a key feature of heart disease but also meds intended to treat it don't work well when NO is insufficiently available. The authors of the study on which the report is based state unequivocally, "In addition, our results point to the possibility that heart failure may represent different clinical conditions depending on NO bioavailability." (6)

According to another report in the journal *Life Sciences* titled "Nitric Oxide and Cardiac Function," NO is a key element in the control of heart contractility. (7) In fact, reduced NO bioavailability imposes an upper limit on myocardial blood flow regulation and its transmural distribution. (8)

4.2.2 Flaxseed Increases NO Bioavailability

Increased NO bioavailability by flaxseed supplementation was reported in the journal *Obesity Medicine* (in the blood vessels of type 2 diabetes patients). The investigators concluded that flaxseeds may offer vasoprotection. (9) Another study published in the *American Journal of Physiology—Heart and Circulation Physiology* concluded that ground flaxseed is rich in L-arginine, and since L-arginine is converted in the vascular endothelium to NO and citrulline, it increases the bioavailability of NO. (1)

4.2.3 Flaxseed Omega-3 Fatty Acid, Alpha-Linolenic Acid, Promotes eNO Formation

It is not solely for antioxidant properties that we value omega-3 polyunsaturated fatty acids, but in addition, a key contribution to cardiovascular function is their promotion of eNO formation: *alpha*-linolenic acid (ALA) improves endothelial function by increasing NO production by directly stimulating eNO synthase gene and protein expression. (10)

Many investigators who tout omega-3 fatty acids for heart health seem unaware of the NO-connection. For instance, in a study titled "The Cardiovascular Effects of Flaxseed and Its Omega-3 Fatty Acid, Alpha-Linolenic Acid" reported in the *Canadian Journal of Cardiology* (used here with permission), we are told,

Preventing the occurrence of cardiovascular disease (CVD) with nutritional interventions is a therapeutic strategy that may warrant greater research attention. The increased use of omega (ω)-3 fatty acids is a powerful example of one such nutritional strategy that may produce significant cardiovascular benefits. Marine food products have provided the traditional dietary sources of ω-3 fatty acids. Flaxseed is an alternative to marine products. It is one of the richest sources of the plant-based ω-3 fatty acid, alpha-linolenic acid (ALA). Based on the results of clinical trials, epidemiological investigations and experimental studies, ingestion of ALA has been suggested to have a positive impact on CVD. Because of its high ALA content, the use of flaxseed has been advocated to combat CVD. (11)

No mention is made of the role of omega-3 in promoting NO synthesis.

The website of the *Institut de Montreal* features an article titled "The Positive Effects of Flaxseed on Cardiovascular Health." The author, Martin Juneau, MD, reports that an average daily intake of 2.2 g of linolenic acid is recommended. This corresponds to one spoon (15 mL) of flaxseed. One needs to grind the seeds to increase absorption of omega-3 fatty acids and allow lignans to transform into active phytoestrogens by intestinal bacteria. However, omega-3 fatty acids are very fragile and sensitive to degradation. Therefore, one should buy whole seeds that can be ground when needed in a simple seed grinder and store the ground seeds in an airtight container in the refrigerator for at least two weeks. He further tells us that the ground seeds have a slightly nutty flavor that goes well with cereals, yogurts and smoothies and can even be used as a salad topping. (12)

Many other studies have reported that flaxseed has recently gained attention in connection with cardiovascular disease because it is the richest known source of both ALA and the phytoestrogen, lignans, as well as being a good source of soluble fiber. Human studies have shown that flaxseed can reduce serum total and low-density lipoprotein cholesterol concentrations, reduce postprandial glucose absorption, decrease some markers of inflammation and raise serum levels of the omega-3 fatty acids, ALA and eicosapentaenoic acid. (13)

4.2.4 Flaxseed Improves the Ejection Fraction

In a study published in the *Journal of Pharmacology and Experimental Therapeutics*, the investigators report that in the *in vivo* myocardial infarction model, secoisolariciresinol diglucoside (SDG) from flaxseed increased capillary density and myocardial function as evidenced by increased fractional shortening and ejection fraction. (14) Fractional shortening is the percentage of size differences of the left ventricle as a measure of how well it is contracting and therefore reducing in size during systole. Values greater than 28% are considered to be normal. SDG is an antioxidant phytoestrogen present in flax, sunflower, sesame and pumpkin seeds.

A year later, these investigators reported in the *Journal of Molecular and Cellular Cardiology* that they observed significant improvement in left ventricular functions in a hypercholesterolemic patient group given SDG (HSDG) as evidenced by increased ejection fraction (55% vs. 45%), fractional shortening (28% vs. 22%) and decreased left ventricular inner diameter in systole (8 mm vs. 6 mm) as compared to a control group (HC). (15)

4.3 ARTERIAL VESSEL COMPLIANCE

During the systole phase of the heartbeat, the heart muscle contracts and pumps blood from the left chamber into the aorta. But the aorta is not devoid of blood. And so the volume of the bolus ejected into the aorta is added to the volume of blood that is still there after the last systole. As a consequence, the vessel momentarily distends—bulges outward, as it were—as shown in Figure 4.2A.

Shortly thereafter, and before the next systole, the wall of the aorta recoils returning the vessel to its previous configuration, as shown in Figure 4.2B.

This successive peristalsic stretch/distention and subsequent recoil pumps blood along in the circulatory system. The sole, albeit by no means lesser role of the heart in blood circulation is the ejection of the bolus from the left ventricle into the blood vessel. The key to how all this works, and therefore the key to blood pressure is "compliance," i.e. the flexibility or distensibility of the vessel wall, i.e. the capacity to distend as a result of pressure from inside and then return to its original shape. Clearly, rigidity such as that due to atherosclerosis and other factors such as those related to aging impair compliance.

Figure 4.3 illustrates the change in a blood vessel due to compliance in normal elastic arteries vs. that in stiff/rigid arteries.

How dependent is arterial compliance on NO? The authors of a study published in the journal *Hypertension* concluded that in human peripheral conduit arteries, the adaptation of smooth muscle *tone* and arterial stiffness during blood flow variations is regulated by the vascular endothelium through the release of eNO. (18) Here again,

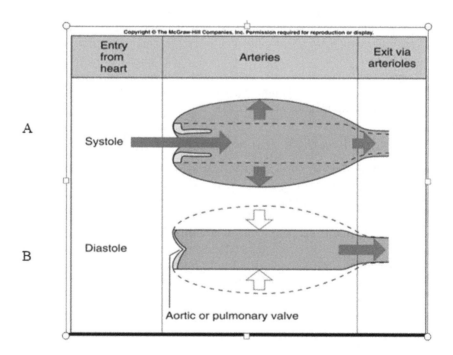

FIGURE 4.2 Distention of the aorta following systole and recoil of the aorta during diastole. [From Serino. (No date) Cardiovascular System: Circulation pathways and BP regulation. https://slideplayer.com/slide/14264710/; accessed 12/15/21. (16) With permission.]

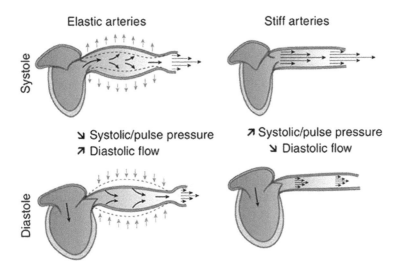

FIGURE 4.3 Schematic representation of the role of arterial compliance (i.e., the inverse of arterial stiffness) in dampening blood pressure pulsatility and assuring adapted blood flow through the peripheral circulation. [(17) Briet, Boutouyrie, Laurent et al. 2012. *Kidney International*. With permission.]

the importance of flaxseed supplementation is emphasized because it is a known NO-donor and without minimizing the antioxidant and other micronutrient constituents properties that benefit blood vessels.

4.3.1 FLAXSEED OIL PROMOTES ARTERIAL BLOOD VESSEL ELASTICITY (COMPLIANCE)

Because the compliance or elasticity of arterial blood vessels diminishes with increasing cardiovascular risk and, conversely, systemic arterial compliance improves through the eating of fish and fish oil, investigators tested the value of high intake of ALA, the plant precursor of fish fatty acids.

Obese people with markers for insulin resistance ate, in turn, four diets of four weeks duration each: saturated/high fat (SHF), alpha-linolenic acid/low fat (ALF), oleic/low fat (OLF) and then SHF again. Daily intake of ALA was 20 grams from margarine products based on flax oil. Systemic arterial compliance was calculated from aortic flow velocity and aortic root driving pressure. Plasma lipids, glucose tolerance and *in vitro* LDL oxidizability were also measured.

Systemic arterial compliance rose significantly with ALF; systemic arterial compliance with OLF was lower than with ALF. Mean arterial blood pressures and results of oral glucose tolerance tests were similar during ALF, OLF and second SHF; total cholesterol levels were also not significantly different. However, insulin sensitivity and high-density lipoprotein (HDL) cholesterol diminished and LDL oxidizability increased with ALF. The marked rise in arterial compliance at least with ALA reflected rapid functional improvement in the systemic arterial circulation despite a rise in LDL oxidizability.

The investigators concluded that dietary omega-3 fatty acids in flax oil improve arterial function. (19)

In the following study, investigators sought to determine the effect of L-arginine on arterial stiffness and oxidative stress in people with chronic kidney disease (CKD): Thirty patients with stage II to IV CKD were administered 9 grams of L-arginine per day orally for a period of 12 weeks.

The parameters evaluated at baseline, at eight weeks, and at the end of 12 weeks were serum nitric oxide (NO), carotid-femoral pulse wave velocity (cf PWV) and radial artery pulse wave analysis, which included aortic augmentation pressure (AP), aortic augmentation index (AIx) at a heart rate of 75 bpm, subendocardial viability ratio, radial pressures and central aortic pressure. Serum levels of NO and malondialdehyde (MDA) were estimated at baseline and at the end of 12 weeks. The control group was composed of age- and sex-matched healthy individuals. Baseline NO levels were low in all the participants.

- *The carotid-femoral pulse wave velocity (cf PWV) is a measure of arterial stiffness determined from the time taken for the arterial pulse to propagate from the carotid to the femoral artery.*
- *The aortic augmentation pressure (AP) is the contribution that wave reflection makes to systolic arterial pressure. It is an indirect measure of arterial stiffness and is calculated as AG divided by pulse pressure (PP) ×100.*
- *The AIx is derived from the aortic pressure waveform and is calculated as aortic augmentation from the initial peak or shoulder to peak pressure divided by pulse pressure.*
- *MDA: Free radicals generate the lipid peroxidation process in an organism. MDA is one of the final products of polyunsaturated fatty acids peroxidation in the cells.*

Administration of L-arginine resulted in improvement in the carotid-radial pulse wave velocity (crPWVr), cf PWV, AIx, AP, and NO. There was no significant change in the levels of MDA.

The investigators concluded that PWV, an indicator of arterial stiffness, is greatly increased even in the early stages of CKD. But supplementation of L-arginine is a safe, well tolerated and effective way of improving endothelial dysfunction in patients with CKD. (20)

Although L-arginine was not derived from flaxseed in the aforementioned study, it is cited in context—i.e., eNO improves arterial blood vessel compliance and other pulse wave parameters. Compliance can be observed indirectly in the *arterial waveform* (see the following section).

4.4 THE ARTERIAL WAVEFORM

The arterial waveform results from the dynamic interactions between the volume of blood ejected by the heart during each beat, the speed with which this volume is ejected by the heart, the ability of the vascular tree to distend and accommodate this ejected volume and the rate at which the ejected volume of blood is able to flow away from the central arterial compartment into the peripheral tissues. (21)

Compliance can be observed as the extent of the "dichrotic notch." The dicrotic notch is a prominent and distinctive feature of the pressure waveform in the central arteries. It is universally used to demarcate the end of systole and the beginning of diastole in these arteries. It is seen as a secondary upstroke in the descending part of a pulse tracing corresponding to the transient increase in aortic pressure when the aortic valve closes.

The arterial pulse waveform can be separated into three distinct components:

- The systolic phase characterized by a rapid increase in pressure to a peak, followed by a rapid decline. This phase begins with the opening of the aortic valve and corresponds to the left ventricular ejection.
- The dicrotic notch, which is widely believed to represent the closure of the aortic valve.
- The diastolic phase, which represents the runoff of blood into the peripheral circulation.

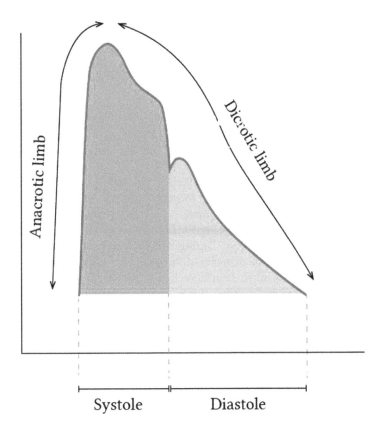

FIGURE 4.4 Arterial pulse waveform over one cardiac cycle. The waveform can be separated into anacrotic (upstroke) and dicrotic (downstroke) limbs. [(22) derangedphysiology.com. With permission.]

However, it is now generally believed that the peripheral dicrotic notch owes more of its shape to the vascular resistance of peripheral vessels, i.e. compliance, than simply as a marker of the closing of the aortic valve.

So we can assess the effectiveness of heart function by estimating the ejection fraction. We can further determine the effectiveness of the arterial vascular system by estimating compliance. In addition, we can assess the status of arterial blood vessels by measuring blood flow. (23) All of these assessment means can be used to evaluate endothelial/endocardial function and the impact of NO deficiency on systemic or regional blood flow. By the same token, they also reflect the benefits of flaxseed supplementation or the benefits of supplementing its constituents singly.

The journal *Physiological Reports* published a clinical study in 2015 titled "Effect of Omega-3 Polyunsaturated Fatty Acid Supplementation on Central Arterial Stiffness and Arterial Wave Reflections in Young and Older Healthy Adults." Based on changes in pulse waveform, the authors concluded that 12 weeks of daily omega-3 supplementation decreases central arterial stiffness (cf PWV) in older adults. (44)

In a clinical study titled "The Effect of L-Arginine on Arterial Stiffness and Oxidative Stress in Chronic Kidney Disease," published in the *Indian Journal of Nephrology* in 2012, the investigators concluded that, based on PWV measures of arterial stiffness, supplementation of L-arginine is a safe, well tolerated and effective way of improving endothelial dysfunction in patients with CKD. (45)

4.5 MEASURING BLOOD FLOW BY FLOW-MEDIATED DILATION (FMD)

One of the most common methods for assessing the effect of raising NO availability is by examining its corresponding effects on regional blood flow. That effect is typically observed in the brachial artery with the method known as flow-mediated dilation (FMD).

FMD is an indirect, noninvasive measure of blood vessel health. The primary cause of FMD is the release of nitric oxide (eNO) by endothelial cells, and in clinical application, there is ultrasound imaging to evaluate brachial artery dilation following a transient period of forearm ischemia.

Here is how the method of observing FMD is described in a report in the *British Journal of Clinical Pharmacology*. During reactive hyperaemia,* induced by cuff inflation and then deflation, the diameter of the artery is measured by high-resolution ultrasound in response to an increase in blood flow causing shear stress. Reactive hyperaemia leads to endothelium-dependent dilatation. The response of the blood vessel is contrasted with the response to sublingual nitroglycerin, an endothelium-independent dilator. The artery is scanned and the diameter measured during two conditions: (1) at baseline, during reactive hyperaemia induced by inflation and then deflation of a sphygmomanometer cuff around the limb, distal to the scanned part of the artery; (2) after administration of sublingual nitroglycerin using a normal antianginal dose of 400 μg, which causes endothelium-independent smooth muscle mediated vasodilatation.

---

* Reactive hyperemia is the excess blood that flows through a blood vessel following the circulation arrest and subsequent restoration of the blood supply. "Hyperaemia" is an archaic form of the word.

It can take between one and ten minutes to obtain a high-quality baseline scan. The cuff inflation period of five minutes was initially decided to produce adequate hyperaemia to allow flow-mediated dilatation, but not to compromise patient comfort. Shorter inflation periods do not seem to produce significant flow-mediated dilatation. The usual scanning period used in their laboratory is 30 seconds before and 90 seconds after the cuff deflation. (24)

FMD compares the response of the brachial artery, after compression to stem blood flow, when given nitroglycerin, a vasodilator substance, and to endothelium-derived NO. Nitroglycerin is a vasodilator because it is a NO-donor. So the test basically asks the question, If I administer a NO-donor, what is the blood vessel response? If I ask the endothelium to supply the NO, how well can it do that by comparison? The description of the previous method is pretty much conventional, but there are published variations in application details.

A study published in the *American Journal of Cardiology* found FMD to be an excellent predictor of long-term adverse cardiovascular events. Participants with below-mean FMD were 278% more likely to experience cardiovascular "events" during the 4.6-year average follow-up period than participants with above-mean FMD. (25) The importance of this information is that it points to the fact that eNO formation is an important clue to cardiovascular health insofar as low eNO availability is an indication of cardiovascular pathophysiology. In addition, enhancing NO formation and availability is now a viable treatment modality both pharmacologically and by nonprescription means.

Does FMD depend on NO? It does. At least to some extent according to a report based on meta-analysis. (26)

4.5.1 Flaxseed and L-Arginine Improve FMD

A number of publications report that flax improves FMD. Keep in mind that FMD is mediated by eNO and thus reflects the patency of endothelial function.

The purpose of a study published in the *European Journal of Clinical Nutrition* was to examine the effect of flaxseed consumption on FMD and inflammatory markers in coronary artery disease (CAD) patients. Fifty patients of both genders with CAD were randomly allocated to 12 weeks consumption of flaxseed (30 grams/day) or usual care control. Before and after the intervention, changes in brachial FMD and plasma high-sensitivity C-reactive protein (hs-CRP),* interleukin-6 (IL-6) and tumor necrosis factor-α (TNF-α) were measured.

It was found that though no significant weight changes were observed in either group, flaxseed consumption resulted in improved FMD. Furthermore, when compared to control participants, flaxseed consumption was associated with reduced inflammatory markers (significant mean change from baseline for hs-CRP, IL-6, and TNF-α). The authors concluded that by adding flaxseed to the diets of CAD patients, it is possible to improve FMD and to lower plasma levels of inflammatory markers. (27)

- *The high-sensitivity C-reactive protein (hs-CRP) test detects lower blood levels of C-reactive protein (CRP), a marker of inflammation.*

- *IL-6, Interleukin 6, is an interleukin that acts as both a proinflammatory cytokine and an anti-inflammatory myokine. It is a multifunctional cytokine that plays a central role in host defense due to its wide range of immune and hematopoietic activities and its potent ability to induce the acute-phase response.*
- *TNF-α, tumor necrosis factor-α, is a cytokine, a small protein used by the immune system for cell signaling. If macrophages detect stressors such as an infection, they release TNF to alert other immune system cells as part of an inflammatory response.*

In a study published in the *Journal of the American College of Nutrition*, the investigators aimed to determine the effects of ALA (from walnuts and flaxseed) on cardiovascular responses to acute stress; FMD of the brachial artery; blood concentrations of endothelin-1, a potent vasoconstrictor encoded by the EDN1 gene and produced by vascular endothelial cells; and arginine-vasopressin (AVP) (an antidiuretic hormone).

The diets significantly reduced diastolic blood pressure and total peripheral resistance, and this effect was evident at rest and during stress. FMD increased by 34% in the diet containing additional ALA. (28) Walnuts, parenthetically, are very high in L-arginine: dried walnuts contain 4.522 grams per cup. One cup of flaxseeds contains about 3.23 grams of L-arginine.

Aging is associated with normal progressive endothelial dysfunction as evidenced by studies of impairment of FMD of the brachial artery. This is a hallmark in the elderly with cardiovascular disease and reduced vascular NO bioavailability. The aim of a study published in the journal *Vascular Medicine*, in 2003, was to determine whether oral L-arginine can improve impaired FMD in healthy very old people.

Healthy participant 73.8 ± 2.7 years old took 8 g p.o. two times daily L-arginine or placebo for 14 days each, separated by a wash-out period of 14 days. It was found that L-arginine significantly improved FMD, whereas the placebo had no effect.

Because NO synthesis can be antagonized by its endogenous inhibitor asymmetric dimethyl L-arginine (ADMA), ADMA plasma concentrations were determined and shown to be elevated at baseline in comparison to healthy middle-aged individuals.

ADMA remained unchanged during treatment, but L-arginine supplementation significantly normalized the L-arginine/ADMA ratio. It was concluded that in healthy very old age endothelial function is impaired and may be improved by oral L-arginine supplementation, probably due to normalization of the L-arginine/ADMA ratio. (46)

ADMA is a naturally occurring metabolic by-product of continual protein modification processes in the cytoplasm of all human cells. Found in blood plasma, it is closely related to L-arginine. ADMA levels rise with "poor" diet/lifestyle, elevated LDL cholesterol, high blood sugar, high blood pressure or smoking—the usual cardiovascular risk suspects.

The Role of Flaxseed Micronutrients in Blood Vessel and Heart Function   79

4.6 ENDOTHELIAL NITRIC OXIDE (eNO) AND CONTROL OF BLOOD PRESSURE

Hypertension is a major risk factor for cardiovascular disease and kidney failure, and reducing elevated blood pressure significantly reduces those risks. Dysfunctional endothelium and reduced bioavailability of NO have been shown in hypertensive individuals to be dependent on the duration and severity of arterial hypertension. (29) Both endothelium-independent and endothelium (NO)-dependent systems control blood pressure and blood flow.

4.6.1 ENDOTHELIUM-INDEPENDENT CONTROL OF BLOOD PRESSURE

In brief, the renin-angiotensin-aldosterone system of the kidneys regulates blood volume. In response to rising blood pressure, the kidneys secrete renin into the blood. Renin converts the plasma protein angiotensinogen into angiotensin I, which in turn is converted into angiotensin II by enzymes from the lungs. Angiotensin II activates two mechanisms that raise blood pressure:

Angiotensin II constricts blood vessels throughout the body, raising blood pressure by increasing resistance to blood flow. Constricted blood vessels reduce the amount of blood delivered to the kidneys, which decreases the kidneys' potential to excrete water, raising blood pressure by increasing blood volume.

Angiotensin II stimulates the adrenal cortex to secrete aldosterone, a hormone that reduces urine output by increasing retention of water and sodium by the kidneys, raising blood pressure by increasing blood volume.

Various substances influence blood pressure: Epinephrine and norepinephrine, which are hormones secreted by the adrenal medulla, raise blood pressure by increasing heart rate and the contractility of the heart muscles and by causing vasoconstriction of arteries and veins.

Antidiuretic hormone produced by the hypothalamus and released by the posterior pituitary raises blood pressure by stimulating the kidneys to retain water, thus raising blood pressure by increasing blood volume.

Atrial natriuretic peptide, a hormone secreted by the atria of the heart, lowers blood pressure by causing vasodilation and by stimulating the kidneys to excrete more water and sodium thus lowering blood pressure by reducing blood volume.

4.6.2 ENDOTHELIUM-DEPENDENT CONTROL OF BLOOD PRESSURE

It is now increasingly evident that endothelial dysfunction, which is characterized by impairment of NO bioavailability, is an important risk factor for hypertension, cardiovascular and kidney disease. NO is a vasodilator that controls blood flow in response to regional blood flow and tissue oxygenation demands.

It has been shown that NO plays a major role in regulating blood pressure and that impaired NO availability can lead to hypertension. Clinical studies have shown that patients with hypertension show reduced arterial vasodilation response to infusion of endothelium-dependent vasodilators such as nitroglycerin and that inhibition of eNO formation raises blood pressure. Impaired NO formation and availability is also implicated in arterial stiffness, a major mechanism of systolic hypertension. (30)

Clearly, NO also regulates resting blood vessel *tone*, adaptation of blood flow to metabolic demand and adaptation of vessel diameter to volume of inflow, i.e., FMD.

> *Vascular "tone" describes the degree of smooth muscle contraction of an arterial blood vessel.*

Arterial hypertension is associated with an increased vascular tone of resistance vessels and a reduced compliance of conduit arteries, along with a thickening of the intima-media leading to vascular "remodeling."

4.6.3 Interaction of Endothelium-Independent and Endothelium-Dependent Blood Flow Control Systems

A review appearing in the journal *Pharmacology and Therapeutics* concludes that endothelium-dependent NO and the autonomic nervous system mechanisms interact in the control of blood flow and in cardiovascular regulation, both in experimental animals and in humans. In fact, NO interacts with the autonomic nervous system both at the central level and peripherally.

The primary effect of NO in humans is a reduction of basal sympathetic vasoconstrictor tone rather than inhibition of the excitability of this system. Impaired NO synthesis in humans, therefore, promotes sustained vasoconstriction by two distinct mechanisms. One is loss of vasodilator tone at vascular smooth muscle cells and the other is by facilitating central neural vasoconstrictor outflow. Insulin resistance, essential hypertension and end-stage renal failure are examples of diseases, where impaired NO buffering of neural outflow may contribute to sustained sympathetic activation.

In addition to the sympathetic nervous system, NO also interacts with the cholinergic nervous system. Cholinergic mechanisms play a major hitherto unrecognized role in offsetting the arterial hypertension and cardiac sympathetic activation caused by inhibition of NO synthesis in normal humans. The investigators concluded that there may be benefits in the use of therapeutic interventions that deliver NO and/or modulate the bioavailability of endogenously produced NO to adjust the autonomic control of the circulation in humans. (31)

Many journal publications conclude, as did the authors of the one cited earlier, that "there may be benefits in the use of therapeutic interventions that deliver NO and/or modulate the bioavailability of endogenously produced NO" to whatever ends. It is becoming increasingly clear that flaxseed *per se*, omega-3 fatty acids, and L-arginine are precisely the interventions they are looking for. These interventions do exactly what they are looking for, i.e., rectify endothelium damage and increase NO bioavailability.

4.6.4 The Role of NO in Vascular Remodeling in Hypertension

Hypertension causes permanent changes in blood vessels, such as vascular remodeling, changes in the structure of resistance vessels contributing to elevated systemic resistance and compliance. Vascular remodeling involves changes in at least four cellular processes: cell growth, cell death, cell migration and the synthesis or degradation of extracellular matrix. It occurs in response to long-standing changes in hemodynamic conditions. (32)

Atherosclerotic narrowing of the arterial lumen is not simply due to enlargement of atherosclerotic lesions. (33) Instead of simply remodeling the narrowed lumen, arteries undergo many changes, such as increasing the outside diameter, to preserve blood flow. This adaptability of the arteries is essential in arterial diseases. As with atherosclerotic coronary disease, peripheral vascular disease and hypertension may be considered a failure of the arterial wall to maintain a suitable mesh size to allow normal blood flow. It has been proposed that the inability of vessels to remodel is a "vascular insufficiency," similar to that observed in the heart during heart failure.

Hypertension elicits two different kinds of diffuse structural changes in the systemic microcirculation. One, "rarefaction," consists of an abnormally low spatial density of arterioles, capillaries and, possibly, venules. The other consists of structural modifications of resistance small arteries and arterioles, which lead to a reduction in lumen diameter and are grouped under the generic name of "remodeling." (34)

While it is well-known that the vascular endothelium mediates the ability of blood vessels to alter their architecture in response to hemodynamic changes, the specific endothelial-derived factors that are responsible for vascular remodeling are unknown. But it is emerging that eNO is a major endothelial-derived mediator controlling vascular remodeling.

For instance, a study in the *Journal of Clinical Investigation* reported that in response to external carotid artery ligation, mice with targeted disruption of the endothelial nitric oxide synthase (eNOS) gene did not remodel their ipsilateral common carotid arteries, whereas wild-type mice did. The eNOS mutant mice displayed a paradoxical increase in wall thickness accompanied by a hyperplastic response of the arterial wall. These findings demonstrate a critical role for endogenous NO as a down regulator of vascular smooth muscle proliferation in response to a remodeling stimulus. Furthermore, the data suggested that a primary defect in the NOS/NO pathway can promote abnormal remodeling and may facilitate pathological changes in vessel wall morphology associated with complex diseases such as hypertension and atherosclerosis. (35)

Likewise, a study published in the journal *Hypertension* concluded that reduced blood flow in hypertensive animals promotes hypertrophy by enhancing smooth muscle cell (SMC) proliferation via mechanisms that reduce the inhibitory effects of NO on SMC proliferation. (36)

NO as a critical regulator of vascular remodeling has also been reported in the journal *Human Genetics '99: The Cardiovascular System*. The authors contend that pharmacologic studies using inhibitors of the enzyme, NOS, have implicated NO as an important endothelial mediator of flow- or pressure-induced arterial remodeling. Long-term treatment of rats with the NOS inhibitor, nitro-l-arginine methyl ester, causes a sustained increase in systemic blood pressure accompanied by marked microvascular remodeling, as judged by an increase in wall-to-lumen ratios of coronary arteries. (37)

In light of the desirability to avoid the notably adverse structural changes of blood vessels in hypertension, maintaining NO bioavailability is of prime concern. That can apparently also be accomplished by flaxseed supplementation in order to supply the substrates L-arginine and cyanogenic glycosides, proven NO-donors. And omega-3 PUFAs can also play a beneficial role:

A review titled "Omega-3 Polyunsaturated Fatty Acids: Structural and Functional Effects on the Vascular Wall" was published in the journal *BioMed Research International* in 2015. The authors contend that by targeting both arterial wall stiffness and endothelial dysfunction, omega-3 PUFAs have the potential to beneficially impact arterial wall remodeling and cardiovascular outcomes. Furthermore, their effects on systemic inflammation, modulation of lipid profile and platelet aggregation are additionally thought to contribute to the reduction of cardiovascular risk. (47)

4.6.5 Flaxseed Combats Hypertension

The purpose of a meta-analysis titled "Flaxseed Consumption May Reduce Blood Pressure: A Systematic Review and Meta-Analysis of Controlled Trials," reported in the *Journal of Nutrition*, was to clarify the effect of flaxseed consumption on blood pressure. The search centered on PubMed (Medline), Cumulative Index to Nursing and Allied Health Literature, and Cochrane Library (Central) through July 2014 for studies in which humans supplemented their habitual diet with flaxseed or its extracts (i.e., oil, lignans, fiber) for ≥ two weeks.

It was found that flaxseed supplementation reduced systolic blood pressure and diastolic blood pressure. These results were not influenced by categorization of participants into higher baseline blood pressure (≥130 mm Hg). An improvement in diastolic blood pressure was observed in subgroup analysis for consuming whole flaxseed and duration of consumption ≥12 weeks.

It was concluded that consumption of flaxseed may lower blood pressure somewhat. The beneficial potential of flaxseed to reduce blood pressure (especially diastolic blood pressure) may be greater when it is consumed as a whole seed and for a duration of >12 weeks. (38)

The purpose of a subsequent study reported in the journal *Hypertension* was to determine the effects of daily consumption of a variety of foods that contained 30 grams of milled flaxseed, or placebo, each day over six months, on systolic blood pressure (SBP) and diastolic blood pressure (DBP) in peripheral artery disease patients. Plasma levels of the omega-3 fatty acid, ALA and enterolignans, increased 2- to 50-fold in the flaxseed-fed group but did not increase significantly in the placebo group.

Patients' body weight was not significantly different between the two groups at any time. After six months, SBP was ≈ 10 mm Hg lower and DBP was ≈ 7 mm Hg lower in the flaxseed group, compared to the placebo.

Patients who entered the trial with an SBP ≥ 140 mm Hg at baseline experienced a significant reduction of 15 mm Hg in SBP, and 7 mm Hg in DBP from flaxseed ingestion. The antihypertensive effect was achieved selectively in hypertensive patients. Circulating ALA levels correlated with SBP and DBP, and lignan levels correlated with changes in DBP.

In summary, flaxseed induced one of the most potent antihypertensive effects achieved by a dietary intervention. (39)

The following meta-analysis published in the journal *Clinical Nutrition* aimed to determine the effects of flaxseed supplements on blood pressure. The search included PUBMED, Cochrane Library, Scopus and Embase up to February 2015 to identify randomized control trials (RCTs) investigating the effect of flaxseed supplements on plasma blood pressure.

It was found that there was a greater effect on both SBP and DBP in the subset of trials with ≥12 weeks of duration vs. the subset lasting <12 weeks. Another subgroup analysis was performed to assess the impact of flaxseed supplement type on blood pressure. Reduction of SBP was significant with flaxseed powder but not oil and lignan extract. However, DBP was significantly reduced with powder and oil preparations but not with lignan extract.

The investigators concluded that this meta-analysis showed significant reductions in both SBP and DBP following supplementation with various flaxseed products. (40)

In a 2020 review titled "The Effects of L-Arginine in Hypertensive Patients: A Literature Review," the authors report a modest decrease in blood pressure with L-arginine supplementation but a greater decrease in blood pressure in hypertensive patients or those with endothelial dysfunction. L-Arginine supplementation has also shown benefits in renal hypertension where there is usually poor endothelial function, a condition that can be recovered by the supplementation of L-arginine. Furthermore, studies show that supplementation of L-arginine improves patients with diabetes mellitus and those with congestive heart failure. (48)

4.7 FLAXSEED COMBATS PERIPHERAL ARTERY DISEASE (PAD)

Peripheral artery disease (PAD) in the legs or lower extremities is the narrowing or blockage of the vessels that carry blood from the heart to the legs. It is primarily caused by the buildup of fatty plaque in the arteries, i.e., atherosclerosis. It should not be surprising to learn that flaxseed is helpful in the treatment of PAD because it had already been shown that so is L-arginine—because it is a NO-donor.

But first, in a report in the journal *Circulation*, investigators tell us that asymmetric dimethylarginine (ADMA) levels are increased in people with hypercholesterolemia, atherosclerosis, hypertension, chronic heart failure, diabetes mellitus and chronic renal failure. In a study published in the journal *Circulation*, investigators report strong evidence for impaired NOS in patients with PAD. ADMA concentrations were notably elevated in their PAD patients. (41) But in a subsequent clinical study, a subgroup of these investigators found that the symptoms of *intermittent claudication* in patients with PAD could be diminished by administration of L-arginine thus improving the condition.

> Intermittent claudication *is pain affecting the calf, and less commonly the thigh and buttock, that is induced by exercise and relieved by rest.*

Patients with intermittent claudication were assigned to receive 2 × 8 grams of L-arginine/day, or 2 × 40 micrograms of prostaglandin E1 (PGE1)/day or no hemodynamically active treatment, for three weeks. The pain-free and absolute walking distances were assessed on a walking 12% slope treadmill at 3 km/h and NO-mediated, FMD of the femoral artery was assessed by ultrasonography at baseline, at one, two and three weeks of therapy and six weeks after the end of treatment.

L-Arginine increased the pain-free walking distance by 230 ± 63% and the absolute walking distance by 155 ± 48%. Prostaglandin E1 improved both parameters by 209 ± 63% and 144 ± 28%, respectively, whereas control patients experienced no significant change. L-Arginine therapy also improved endothelium-dependent vasodilation in the femoral artery (FMD), whereas PGE1 had no such effect.

There was a significant linear correlation between the L-arginine/ADMA ratio and the pain-free walking distance at baseline. L-Arginine treatment elevated the plasma L-arginine/ADMA ratio and increased urinary nitrate and cyclic GMP excretion rates, indicating normalized endogenous NO formation. Prostaglandin E1 therapy had no significant effect on any of these parameters. The investigators concluded that restoring NO formation and endothelium-dependent vasodilation by L-arginine improves the clinical symptoms of intermittent claudication in patients with peripheral arterial disease. (42)

> *Prostaglandin E1, Alprostadil, a medication, is used as a smooth muscle relaxant and vasodilator.*

A number of clinical studies support the beneficial effects of flaxseed and its constituents in PAD. For instance, there is enough interest in its possible benefits in PAD to even warrant an ongoing trial called FLAX-PAD reported in the journal *Contemporary Clinical Trials* in 2011. However, so far we know only from that trial that in PAD patients fed 30 g of milled flaxseed every day for six months, blood pressure dropped significantly. (49)

There is a school of thought that a number of cardiovascular disorders are in fact omega-3 deficiency diseases. A recent study reported that individuals diagnosed with PAD have a lower Omega-3 Index compared to those who don't have that disease. The study titled "Peripheral Artery Disease Is Associated with a Deficiency of Erythrocyte Membrane n-3 Polyunsaturated Fatty Acids" was published in the journal *Lipids* in 2019. (50)

The omega index is a measure of erythrocyte (red blood cells) membrane omega-3 concentration as a percentage of total fatty acids. (51)

There are clinical studies on the effects of L-arginine supplementation in PAD. Some support supplementation while others don't. One of the "don'ts" is titled "Nitric Oxide in Peripheral Arterial Insufficiency—NO-PAIN" (June 28, 2007). It appears on the website of the American College of Cardiology (ACC) (www.acc.org/latest-in-cardiology/clinical-trials/2010/02/23/19/12/nopain; accessed 1/19/22). It reports a trial that aimed to determine the effect of long-term therapy with oral L-arginine on vascular reactivity and functional capacity in patients with intermittent claudication due to PAD. It was found that the patients actually got *worse* on 3 g per day of oral L-arginine for six months.

According to a report titled "Variations in L-arginine Intake According to Demographic Characteristics and Cardiovascular Risk," published in the journal *Nutrition Research* in 2008, the average dietary L-arginine intake for the US adult population is 4.40 g/day. A daily dosage of oral L-arginine of 3 grams is less than the average American consumes in meals daily. Typical clinical dosages hover around 9 g/day. (52)

The Mayo Clinic website recommends L-arginine for PAD (www.mayoclinic.org/drugs-supplements-l-arginine/art-20364681; accessed 1/19/22). But it does not say how much one should take.

Here is a study that seemed to have somewhat better success: In a pilot study of L-arginine supplementation on functional capacity in peripheral arterial disease published in the journal *Vascular Medicine*, in 2005, patients were assigned to oral doses of 0, 3, 6 or 9 g of L-arginine daily in three divided doses for 12 weeks. No significant differences were observed in absolute claudication distance between the treatment and the control groups. However, a trend was observed for a greater increase in walking distance in the group treated with 3 g L-arginine daily, and there was a trend for an improvement in walking speed in patients treated with L-arginine. (53)

4.8 SUMMARY

Endothelium-derived nitric oxide (eNO), an intrinsic vasodilator, is essential to the control of blood flow and heart function. It is ordinarily derived in the body from the amino acid L-arginine. eNO deficiency is implicated in blood vessel compliance and heart and blood vessel diseases, including PAD. Supplementing L-arginine has been clinically proven to correct deficiency and restore function. But supplementing flaxseed has likewise proven clinically effective in treating blood vessel and heart diseases because, like L-arginine, it is a NO-donor.

4.9 REFERENCES

1. Parikh M, Netticadan T, and GN Pierce. 2018. Flaxseed: Its bioactive components and their cardiovascular benefits. *American Journal of Physiology—Heart and Circulation Physiology*, Feb 1; 314(2): H146–H159. DOI:10.1152/ajpheart.00400.2017.
2. www.mayoclinic.org/diseases-conditions/heart-failure/symptoms-causes/syc-20373142; accessed 3/28/19.
3. Kellym RA, Balligand J-L, and TW Smith. 1996. Nitric oxide and cardiac function. *Circulation Research*, Sep; 79(3): 363–380. DOI:10.1161/01.RES.79.3.363.
4. Cai H, Li Z, Goette A, Mera F, Honeycutt C, Feterik K, Wilcox JN, Dudley SC, Harrison DG, and JJ Langberg. 2002. Downregulation of endocardial nitric oxide synthase expression and nitric oxide production in atrial fibrillation: Potential mechanisms for atrial thrombosis and stroke. *Circulation*, Nov; 106(22): 2854–2858. DOI:10.1161/01.CIR.0000039327.11661.16.
5. www.sciencedaily.com/releases/2018/05/180514132501.htm.
6. Hayashi H, Hess DT, Zhang R, Sugi K, Gao H, Tan BL, Bowles DE, Milano CA, Jain MK, Koch WJ, and JS Stamler. 2018. S-Nitrosylation of β-Arrestins biases receptor signaling and confers ligand independence. *Molecular Cell*, May 3; 70(3): 473–487. DOI:10.1016/j.molcel.2018.03.034.
7. Rastaldo R, Pagliaro P, Cappello S, Penna C, Mancardi D, Westerhof N, and G Losano. 2007. Nitric oxide and cardiac function. *Life Sciences*, Aug 16; 81(10): 779–793. DOI:10.1016/j.lfs.2007.07.019.

8. Kingma JG Jr, Simard D, and JR Rouleau. 2015. Nitric oxide bioavailability affects cardiovascular regulation dependent on cardiac nerve status. *Autonomic Neuroscience*, Jan; 187: 70–75. DOI:10.1016/j.autneu.2014.11.003.
9. Ricklefs-Johnson K, Johnston CS, and KL Sweazea. 2017. Ground flaxseed increased nitric oxide levels in adults with type 2 diabetes: A randomized comparative effectiveness study of supplemental flaxseed and psyllium fiber. *Obesity Medicine*, Mar; 5: 16–24. DOI:10.1016/j.obmed.2017.01.002.
10. Zanetti M, Grillo A, Losurdo P, Panizon E, Mearelli F, Cattin L, Barazzoni R, and R Carretta. 2015. Omega-3 polyunsaturated fatty acids: Structural and functional effects on the vascular wall. *BioMed Research International*, 2015: 791978. DOI:10.1155/2015/791978.
11. Rodriguez-Leyva D, Bassett CMC, McCullough R, and GN Pierce. 2010. The cardiovascular effects of flaxseed and its omega-3 fatty acid, alpha-linolenic acid. *Canadian Journal of Cardiology*, Nov; 26(9): 489–496. DOI:10.1016/s0828-282x(10)70455-4.
12. Juneau M. 2018. *The positive effects of flaxseed on cardiovascular health*. https://observatoireprevention.org/en/2018/01/25/the-positive-effects-of-flaxseed-on-cardiovascular-health/; accessed 10/27/21.
13. Bloedon LeAT, and PO Szapary. 2004. Flaxseed and cardiovascular risk. *Nutrition Reviews*, Jan; 62(1): 18–27. DOI:10.1111/j.1753-4887.2004.tb00002.x.
14. Penumathsa SV, Koneru S, Thirunavukkarasu M, Zhan L, Prasad K, and N Maulik. 2007. Secoisolariciresinol diglucoside: Relevance to angiogenesis and cardioprotection against ischemia-reperfusion injury. *Journal of Pharmacology and Experimental Therapeutics*, 320: 951–959. DOI:10.1124/jpet.106.114165.
15. Penumathsa SV, Koneru S, Zhan L, John S, Menon VP, Prasad K, and N Maulik. 2008. Secoisolariciresinol diglucoside induces neovascularization-mediated cardioprotection against ischemia-reperfusion injury in hypercholesterolemic myocardium. *Journal of Molecular and Cellular Cardiology*, 44: 170–179. DOI:10.1016/j.yjmcc.2007.09.014.
16. Serino T. No date. *Cardiovascular system: Circulation pathways and BP regulation*. https://slideplayer.com/slide/14264710/; accessed 12/15/21.
17. Briet M, Boutouyrie P, Laurent S, and GM London. 2012. Arterial stiffness and pulse pressure in CKD and ESRD. *Kidney International*, Aug; 82(4): 388–400. DOI:10.1038/ki.2012.131.
18. Bellien J, Favre J, Iacob M, Gao J, Thuillez C, Richard V, and R Joannidès. 2010. Arterial stiffness is regulated by nitric oxide and endothelium-derived hyperpolarizing factor during changes in blood flow in humans. *Hypertension*, Jan 18; 55(3): 674–680. DOI:10.1161/HYPERTENSIONAHA.109.142190.
19. Nestel PJ, Pomeroy SE, Sasahara T, Yamashita T, Liang YL, Dart AM, Jennings JL, Abbey M, and JD Cameron.1997. Arterial compliance in obese subjects is improved with dietary plant n-3 fatty acid from flaxseed oil despite increased LDL oxidizability. *Arteriosclerosis, Thrombosis, and Vascular Biology*, Jun; 17(6): 1163–1170. DOI:10.1161/01.atv.17.6.1163.
20. Annavarajula SK, Dakshinamurty KV, Naidu MUR, and CP Reddy. 2012. The effect of L-arginine on arterial stiffness and oxidative stress in chronic kidney disease. *Indian Journal of Nephrology*, Sep–Oct; 22(5): 340–346. DOI:10.4103/0971-4065.103907.
21. Nirmalan M, and PM Dark. 2014. Broader applications of arterial pressure wave form analysis. *Continuing Education in Anaesthesia Critical Care and Pain*, Dec; 14(6): 285–290. DOI:10.1093/bjaceaccp/mkt078.
22. Yartsev A. 2015. *Deranged physiology. Normal arterial line waveforms*. https://derangedphysiology.com/main/cicm-primary-exam/required-reading/cardiovascular-system/Chapter%20760/normal-arterial-line-waveforms; accessed 10/26/21.
23. Chien J-C, Wang J-P, Hsueh M-L, Cheng P-S, and F-C Chong. 2005. An effective image measurement in brachial flow-mediated dilation response analysis. *Computer Science*,

Medicine. Published in IEEE Engineering in Medicine, pp. 1750–1753. DOI:10.1109/IEMBS.2005.1616784.
24. Raitakari OT, and DS Celermajer. 2000. Flow-mediated dilatation. *British Journal of Clinical Pharmacology*, Nov; 50(5): 397–404. DOI:10.1046/j.1365-2125.2000.00277.x.
25. Shechter MM, Shechter A, Koren-Morag N, Feinberg MS, and L Hiersch. 2014. Usefulness of brachial artery flow-mediated dilation to predict long-term cardiovascular events in subjects without heart disease. *American Journal of Cardiology*, Jan 1; 113(1): 162–167. DOI:10.1016/j.amjcard.2013.08.051.
26. Green DJ, Dawson EA, Groenewoud HMM, Jones H, and DHJ Thijssen. 2014. Is flow-mediated dilation nitric oxide mediated? A meta-analysis. *Hypertension*, 63: 376–382. DOI:10.1161/HYPERTENSIONAHA.113.02044.
27. Khandouzi N, Zahedmehr A, Mohammadzadeh A, Sanati HR, and J Nasrollahzadeh. 2019. Effect of flaxseed consumption on flow-mediated dilation and inflammatory biomarkers in patients with coronary artery disease: A randomized controlled trial. *European Journal of Clinical Nutrition*, Feb; 73(2): 258–265. DOI:10.1038/s41430-018-0268-x.
28. West SG, Krick AL, Klein LC, Zhao G, Wojtowicz TF, McGuiness M, Bagshaw DM, Wagner P, Ceballos RM, Holub BJ, and PM Kris-Etherton. 2010. Effects of diets high in walnuts and flax oil on hemodynamic responses to stress and vascular endothelial function. *Journal of the American College of Nutrition*, Dec; 29(6): 595–603. PMCID: PMC3862179; NIHMSID: NIHMS418149.
29. Kelm M. 2003. The L-arginine-nitric oxide pathway in hypertension. *Current Hypertension Reports*, Feb; 5(1): 80–86. DOI:10.1007/s11906-003-0015-z.
30. Hermann M, Flammer A, and TF Lüscher. 2006. Nitric oxide in hypertension. *Journal of Clinical Hypertension (Greenwich)*, Dec; 8(12 Suppl 4): 17–29. DOI:10.1111/j.1524-6175.2006.06032.x.
31. Sartori C, Lepori M, and U Scherrer. 2005. Interaction between nitric oxide and the cholinergic and sympathetic nervous system in cardiovascular control in humans. *Pharmacology and Therapeutics*, May; 106(2): 209–220. DOI:10.1016/j.pharmthera.2004.11.009.
32. Gibbons GH, and VJ Dzau. 1994. The emerging concept of vascular remodeling. *New England Journal of Medicine*, May; 330: 1431–1438. DOI:10.1056/NEJM199405193302008.
33. Glagov S, Weisenberg E, Zarins CK, Stankunavicius R, and GJ Kolettis. 1987. Compensatory enlargement of human atherosclerotic coronary arteries. *New England Journal of Medicine*, May; 316: 1371–1375. DOI:10.1056/NEJM198705283162204.
34. Renna NF, de las Heras N, and RM Miatello. 2013. Pathophysiology of vascular remodeling in hypertension. *International Journal of Hypertension*, Jul; 2013(Article ID 808353): 7 DOI:10.1155/2013/808353.
35. Rudic RD, Shesely EG, Maeda N, Smithies O, Segal SS, and WC Sessa. 1998. Direct evidence for the importance of endothelium-derived nitric oxide in vascular remodeling. *Journal of Clinical Investigation*, Feb 15; 101(4): 731–736. DOI:10.1172/JCI1699.
36. Ueno H, Kanellakis P, Agrotis A, and A Bobik. 2000. Blood flow regulates the development of vascular hypertrophy, smooth muscle cell proliferation, and endothelial cell nitric oxide synthase in hypertension. *Hypertension*, Jul; 36(1): 89–96. DOI:10.1161/01.hyp.36.1.89.
37. Numaguchi K, Egashira K, Takemoto M, Kadokami T, Shimokawa H, Sueishi K, and A Takeshita. 1995. Chronic inhibition of nitric oxide synthesis causes coronary microvascular remodeling in rats. *Hypertension*, Dec; 26(6 Pt 1): 957–962. DOI:10.1161/01.hyp.26.6.957.
38. Khalesi S, Irwin C, and M Schubert. 2015. Flaxseed consumption may reduce blood pressure: A systematic review and meta-analysis of controlled trials. *Journal of Nutrition*, Apr; 145(4): 758–765. DOI:10.3945/jn.114.205302.

39. Rodriguez-Leyva D, Weighell W, Edel AL, LaVallee R, Dibrov E, Pinneker R, Maddaford TG, Ramjiawan B, Aliani M, Guzman R, and GN Pierce. 2013. Potent antihypertensive action of dietary flaxseed in hypertensive patients. *Hypertension*, Dec; 62(6): 1081–1089. DOI:10.1161/Hypertensionaha.113.02094.
40. Ursoniu S, Sahebkar A, Andrica F, Serban C, and M Banach. 2016. Effects of flaxseed supplements on blood pressure: A systematic review and meta-analysis of controlled clinical trial. Lipid and blood pressure meta-analysis Collaboration (LBPMC) Group. *Clinical Nutrition* (Edinburgh, Scotland), Jun; 35(3): 615–625. DOI:10.1016/j.clnu.2015.05.012.
41. Böger RH, Bode-Böger SM, Thiele W, Junker W, Alexander K, and JC Frölich. 1997. Biochemical evidence for impaired nitric oxide synthesis in patients with peripheral arterial occlusive disease. *Circulation*, Apr 15; 95(8): 2068–2074. DOI:10.1161/01.cir.95.8.2068. PMID: 91335.
42. Böger RH, Bode-Böger SM, Thiele W, Creutzig A, Alexander K, and JC Frölich. 1998. Restoring vascular nitric oxide formation by L-arginine improves the symptoms of intermittent claudication in patients with peripheral arterial occlusive disease. *Journal of the American College of Cardiology*, Nov; 32(5): 1336–1344. DOI:10.1016/s0735-1097(98)00375-1.
43. Kang J-S. 2020. Dietary restriction of amino acids for cancer therapy. *Nutrition and Metabolism*, 17(20). DOI:10.1186/s12986-020-00439-x.
44. Monahan KD, Feehan RP, Blaha C, and DJ McLaughlin. 2015. Effect of omega-3 polyunsaturated fatty acid supplementation on central arterial stiffness and arterial wave reflections in young and older healthy adults. *Physiological Reports*, Jun; 3(6): e12438. DOI:10.14814/phy2.12438.
45. Annavarajula SK, Dakshinamurty KV, Naidu MUR, and C Prabhakar Reddy. 2012. The effect of L-arginine on arterial stiffness and oxidative stress in chronic kidney disease. *Indian Journal of Nephrology*, Sep–Oct; 22(5): 340–346. DOI:10.4103/0971-4065.103907.
46. Bode-Böger SM, Muke JX, Surdacki A, Brabant G, Böger RH, and JC Frölich. 2003. Oral L-arginine improves endothelial function in healthy individuals older than 70 years. *Vascular Medicine*, May; 8(2): 77–81. DOI:10.1191/1358863x03vm474oa.
47. Zanetti M, Grillo A, Losurdo P, Panizon E, Mearelli F, Cattin L, Barazzoni R, and R Carretta. 2015. Omega-3 polyunsaturated fatty acids: Structural and functional effects on the vascular wall. *BioMed Research International*, Aug 2; 2015: 791978. DOI:10.1155/2015/791978.
48. Abukhodair AW, Abukhudair W, and MS Alqarni. 2021. The effects of L-arginine in hypertensive atients: A literature review. *Cureus*, Dec 17; 13(12): e20485. DOI:10.7759/cureus.20485.
49. Leyva DR, Zahradka P, Ramjiawan B, Guzman R, Aliani M, and GN Pierce. 2011. The effect of dietary flaxseed on improving symptoms of cardiovascular disease in patients with peripheral artery disease: Rationale and design of the FLAX-PAD randomized controlled trial. *Contemporary Clinical Trials*, Sep; 32(5): 724–730. DOI:10.1016/j.cct.2011.05.005.
50. Ramirez JL, Zahner GJ, Spaulding KA, Khetani SA, Hills NK, Gasper WJ, Harris WS, Cohen BE, and SM Grenon. 2019. Peripheral artery disease is associated with a deficiency of erythrocyte membrane n-3 polyunsaturated fatty acids. *Lipids*, Apr; 54(4): 211–219. DOI:10.1002/lipd.12140.
51. Harris WS, and C von Schacky. 2004. The omega-3 index: A new risk factor for death from coronary heart disease? *Preventive Medicine*, Jul; 39(1): 212–220. DOI:10.1016/j.ypmed.2004.02.030.
52. King DE, Mainous AG, and ME Geesey. 2008. Variations in L-arginine intake according to demographic characteristics and cardiovascular risk. *Nutrition Research*, Jan; 28(1): 21–24. DOI:10.1016/j.nutres.2007.11.003.
53. Oka RK, Szuba A, Giacomini JC, and JP Cooke. 2005. A pilot study of L-arginine supplementation on functional capacity in peripheral arterial disease. *Vascular Medicine*, 10: 265–274.

5 Omega-3 Fatty Acids and NO from Flax Intervention in Atherosclerosis and Chronic Systemic Inflammation

5.1 ATHEROSCLEROSIS

Atherosclerosis is a life-threatening predominantly asymptomatic pandemic condition, a known health hazard that is responsible for more annual deaths in the United States than COVID-19. It is the thickening, and therefore hardening, of the arteries caused by a buildup of plaque in the blood vessel wall. A lipoprotein-driven disease, it leads to plaque formation at specific sites of the arterial tree through intimal inflammation, necrosis, fibrosis and calcification. It is said to lead to hypertension, heart disease and peripheral vascular disease.

Atherosclerosis is concerning because it causes clinical diseases by obstructing blood flow to the heart (coronary heart disease), to the brain (stroke) or to lower extremities.

After decades of relatively slow progression, atheromas (plaques) may suddenly cause life-threatening thrombosis. Most often, the culprit is blood vessel wall rupture with exposure of highly thrombogenic red cell–rich necrotic core material (see Figure 5.1). What sets the stage for this to occur is an extremely thin fibrous cap, a layer of fibrous connective tissue that is thicker and less cellular than the normal intima, containing macrophages and smooth muscle cells.

However, the mechanisms involved in plaque erosion remain largely unknown, although coronary artery spasm is suspected. (1) Figure 5.1 summarizes how medicine generally understands the nature of atherosclerosis, and it forms the basis for treatment recommendations. In the figure, VSMCs stands for vascular smooth muscle cells, and EC stands for endothelial cell.

Figure 5.1 illustrates atherosclerosis and unstable atherosclerotic plaque in aging.

The emphasis is on the rupture of the arterial wall leading to thrombosis. But though there is no mention of it in that publication, and it is quite apparent in the illustration, there is another very important aspect of atherosclerosis: Long before it causes overt cardiovascular and related diseases, it progressively damages the

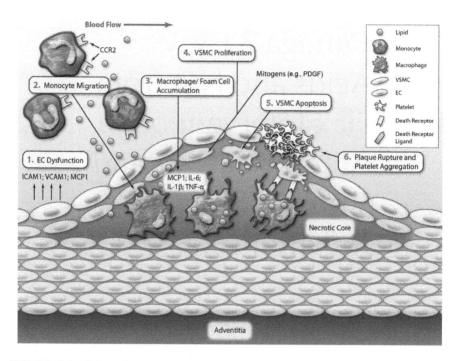

FIGURE 5.1 Schematic of atherogenesis and an unstable atherosclerotic plaque. The advanced atherosclerotic plaque consists of a fibrous cap rich in VSMCs and collagen, surrounding a "necrotic" core comprising lipids, foam cells and debris. Plaque formation involves a series of events initiated from (1) EC dysfunction and activation with increased surface adhesion molecules on ECs, including ICAM-1 and VCAM-1, and augmented vascular permeability promoting the (2) attachment and infiltration of lipid and inflammatory cells into the subendothelial space. (3) Monocytes differentiate into macrophages, engulf lipid to form foam cells and release proinflammatory cytokines (e.g., MCP1, IL-6, IL-1β) to create an inflammatory environment. (4) In early lesions, VSMCs proliferate/migrate in response to mitogens such as platelet-derived growth factor (PDGF) and synthesize collagen to form the fibrous cap that encloses the growing lipid core. At later stages, VSMCs undergo senescence and release multiple cytokines as part of the senescence-associated secretory phenotype, which augments the preexisting inflammation. (5) The gradual loss of VSMCs by apoptosis, in part mediated by engagement of death receptors on VSMCs with death ligands on macrophages and T lymphocytes, and increased activity of matrix-degrading enzymes in the cap result in (6) plaque rupture, with subsequent platelet attachment and thrombosis. Each of the processes involved in atherogenesis and plaque rupture indicated as (1) to (6) are promoted by cellular senescence. (Illustration: Cosmocyte/Ben Smith.) [(2) Wang and Bennett. 2012. Aging and atherosclerosis. Mechanisms, functional consequences, and potential therapeutics for cellular senescence. *Circulation Research*, Jul 6; 111(2): 111:245–259. https://doi.org/10.1161/CIRCRESAHA.111.261388.]

endothelium. The "necrotic core" distances the endothelium from its blood supply, the internal longitudinal *vasa vasorum* (not shown), thus damaging it and impairing regional eNO formation. What's more, as plaque forms, atherosclerosis causes inflammation of the *vasa vasorum*. (3) Inflammation impairs NO formation by the *vasa vasorum*, on which both the arterial blood vessel and the *vasa vasorum* actually depend, and that also facilitates migration of monocytic cells to sites of early disease. (4)

It is also generally understood that diet and lifestyle factors play a key role in atherosclerosis. The emphasis is usually on saturated fats in the diet and on alcohol use, smoking and physical inactivity. But there is now a common understanding that atherosclerosis is an inflammatory disease, and there is substantial scientific literature on the role of reactive oxygen species (ROS) in plaque formation, and these arise largely from mitochondria metabolic activity. In fact, ROS have been shown to promote atherosclerotic plaque formation. (5)

In fact, investigators contend, in an article published in the journal *Molecular Nutrition* and Food Research in 2005, that diet-derived oxidized fatty acids in the chylomicron remnants formed in the intestine that transport dietary triglyceride to peripheral tissues and cholesterol to the liver, as well as LDL, accelerate atherosclerosis by increasing oxidized lipid levels in circulating LDL and chylomicron remnants.

This hypothesis is supported by feeding experiments on animals. When rabbits were fed oxidized fatty acids or oxidized cholesterol, the fatty streak lesions in the aorta were increased by 100%. Moreover, dietary oxidized cholesterol significantly increased aortic lesions in apo-E and LDL receptor-deficient mice.

A typical Western Diet is rich in oxidized fats and therefore could contribute to the increased arterial atherosclerosis in our population. (6) In a 1997 animal-model (rabbits) study titled "Dietary Flax Seed in Prevention of Hypercholesterolemic Atherosclerosis," published in the journal *Atherosclerosis*, the investigator concluded that because of its antioxidant activity, *"flax seed supplementation is effective in reducing hypercholesterolemic atherosclerosis markedly without lowering serum cholesterol."* (7)

The implication of this study is that concerning atherosclerosis, it is not simply a matter of amassing serum cholesterol but whether it is or it is not oxidized. Flaxseed and flax oil antioxidant constituents have been shown to even reverse atherosclerosis progression (8) and that is now becoming increasingly well-known, albeit not yet mainstream.

In part, this may be because some of the most convincing studies are conducted on animal models—rabbits, usually. This, despite the fact that this animal model is conventional in trials on prescription drugs—like statins—used to combat atherosclerosis. Rabbits are subject to diet-induced atherosclerosis just as we are, and they respond to anti-atherosclerosis therapy in a way similar to the way that we do.

In a study published in the *American Journal of Physiology. Heart and Circulatory Physiology* in 2013, investigators aimed to determine the therapeutic potential of dietary flaxseed on atherosclerotic plaque regression and vascular contractile function in a rabbit model. Rabbits received either a regular diet for 12 weeks (group I) or a 1% cholesterol-supplemented diet for four weeks, followed by a regular diet for eight weeks (group II).

The remaining experimental animals were treated as in group II but were fed for an additional 14 weeks with either a regular diet (group III) or a 10% flaxseed-supplemented diet (group IV).

Animals in group II showed clear evidence of plaque growth stabilization. Their vessels also exhibited significantly lower norepinephrine-induced contraction and an impaired relaxation response to acetylcholine compared with animals in group I. Dietary flaxseed supplementation resulted in a significant ≈40% reduction in plaque formation. Animals in both groups III and IV displayed improved contraction and endothelium-dependent vessel relaxation. (9)

5.1.1 THE CAUSAL ROLE OF ROS IN ATHEROSCLEROSIS

According to a report published in the journal *Arteriosclerosis, Thrombosis, and Vascular Biology* in 2017, excessive concentrations of lipids result in free radical formation, and interaction of these molecules with the endothelial wall of the arteries leads to endothelial inflammation. An inflamed endothelium recruits inflammatory cells such as monocytes via the expression of various mediators and chemokines. (10) This in addition to the imbalance of ROS generation leads to monocytes becoming foam cells that consume dead cells and lipids.

This debris eventually develops into a sclerotic fibrofatty plaque, which decreases the compliance of the vessel, increases the possibility of embolus or thrombus development through plaque rupture and, finally, increases the risk of multiple comorbidities. (11) In all of these processes, ROS play a significant role in homeostasis of vascular cells and the pathogenesis of atherosclerosis. (12)

A review published in the journal *Frontiers in Cardiovascular Medicine* in 2019 concludes that subclinical nonatherosclerotic intimal lesions emerge before the appearance of pathologic intimal thickening and advanced atherosclerotic plaques. Intimal thickening is associated with several risk factors, including oxidative stress due to ROS, inflammatory cytokines and lipids. The main ROS producing system *in vivo* is reduced nicotinamide adenine dinucleotide phosphate (NADPH) oxidase (Nox). (13)

The previous finding was corroborated in a review published in the journal *Antioxidants* in 2017 in which the investigators also report that the major source of ROS generated within the vascular system is the NADPH oxidase family of enzymes (Nox), of which seven members have been characterized.

The Nox family are critical determinants of the redox state within the vessel wall that dictate, in part, the pathophysiology of several vascular phenotypes.* The journal articles cited highlight the putative role of ROS in controlling what happens to blood vessels by promoting endothelial dysfunction, altering vascular smooth muscle phenotype and adversely altering vascular stem cells. (14)

---

* The phenotype is the observable traits, such as height, eye color and blood type. The genetic contribution to the phenotype is called the genotype.

5.1.2 OMEGA-3 FATTY ACIDS, AN ANTIOXIDANT FLAXSEED CONSTITUENT CAN PREVENT, EVEN REVERSE, ATHEROSCLEROSIS

Omega–3 fatty acids, also called omega-3 oils, ω–3 fatty acids or n–3 fatty acids, are polyunsaturated fatty acids (PUFAs) found in foods, such as fish and seeds, and in dietary supplements, such as fish oil. The three main omega-3 fatty acids are

- Alpha-linolenic acid (ALA)
- Eicosapentaenoic acid (EPA)
- Docosahexaenoic acid (DHA)

ALA is found mainly in plant oils such as flaxseed, soybean, and canola oils. DHA and EPA are found in fish—oily fish such as salmon and mackerel, in particular—and other seafood. It is an essential fatty acid—the body can't make it—and it must be obtained from the foods and beverages we consume. The body can convert some ALA into EPA and then to DHA, but only in very small amounts. Therefore, getting EPA and DHA from foods and dietary supplements is the only practical way to increase levels of these omega-3 fatty acids in the body. Omega-3s are important components of cell membranes.

Consuming flaxseed can provide ALA to the circulation and tissues of the body. But what is the human requirement for omega-3 PUFAs? One source recommended a daily intake of 2.22 grams of ALA based on a 2,000 kcal diet. (15) ALA levels rise as soon as two weeks after the initiation of flaxseed supplementation. (16)

The bioavailability of ALA is dependent on the type of flax. Golden flaxseeds have more PUFAs and less monounsaturated fatty acids compared to brown flaxseeds. They also have larger amounts of the two essential fats that your body isn't able to produce: ALA and linoleic acid. ALA has greater bioavailability in oil than in milled seed and has greater bioavailability in milled seed than in whole seed. (17)

Crushing and milling of flaxseed substantially improve the bioavailability of enterolignans (18) likely due to the improved accessibility of the colon bacteria to crushed and ground flaxseed, the dose of flaxseed ingested (19) and the fat composition of the diet. Concurrent administration of linoleic acid (AKA omega-6, LA) in the diet will reduce ALA accumulation (19) because of competition among the enzymes involved in the elongation and desaturation of LA and ALA. EPA and DHA are more rapidly incorporated into plasma and membrane lipids and produce more rapid effects than ALA.

Average daily recommended amounts for ALA in grams (g) are listed in Table 5.1

A ratio of alpha-linoleic acid (LA) to ALA of 4:1 or lower is optimal for the elongation of 11 grams of ALA to 1 gram of long-chain omega-3 PUFAs. (20) Age does not appear to influence ALA bioavailability or its conversion to DHA. (21)

5.1.3 OMEGA-3 FATTY ACIDS FROM FLAXSEED

Flaxseed is one of the richest plant sources of the omega-3 fatty ALA. The omega-3 fatty acids found in flaxseed differ from those in fish. The health benefits of fish oil are believed to derive principally from two omega-3 fats, eico-sapenta-enoic acid

TABLE 5.1
Recommended amount of ALA by age and gender

Life Stage	Recommended Amount of ALA
Birth to 12 months*	0.5 g
Children 1–3 years	0.7 g
Children 4–8 years	0.9 g
Boys 9–13 years	1.2 g
Girls 9–13 years	1.0 g
Teen boys 14–18 years	1.6 g
Teen girls 14–18 years	1.1 g
Pregnant teens and women	1.4 g
Breastfeeding teens and women	1.3 g

Source: ods.od.nih.gov.
*As total omega-3s. All other values are for ALA alone.

(EPA) and doco-sahexa-enoic acid (DHA) [hyphens inserted here to help pronunciation]. Flaxseed, on the other hand, contains a third, plant-based omega-3 ALA. The typical North American diet provides approximately 1.4 grams of ALA per day and 0.1 gram to 0.2 grams of EPA and DHA. (22)

A study published in the *American Journal of Clinical Nutrition* in 2006, concerned plasma phospholipid omega-3 fatty acid concentrations after ALA supplementation. It was reported that ALA supplementation with up to 14 grams/day resulted in dose-dependent (but modest) increases in plasma ALA concentrations. Some of the observed variability, especially at low ALA doses, was attributed to differences in the amount of omega-6 linoleic acid (LA) concurrently in the diet. The dose response appeared linear. There were small increases in EPA after ALA supplementation; however, plasma phospholipid DHA, an essential omega-3 fatty acid, concentrations were not observed to increase. (19)

5.1.4 Omega-3 Fatty Acids from Flaxseed and Elevated Blood Cholesterol

Many studies have reported the beneficial effects of flaxseed on normalizing blood total cholesterol (TC), on LDL cholesterol or on high-density lipoprotein (HDL) cholesterol. For instance, in 1997, an article published in the journal *Arteriosclerosis, Thrombosis and Vascular Biology* concluded, "*The marked rise in arterial compliance at least with α-linolenic acid reflected rapid functional improvement in the systemic arterial circulation despite a rise in LDL oxidizability. Dietary n-3 fatty acids in flax oil thus confer a novel approach to improving arterial function.*" (23)

Investigators reported in 2008, in the *Journal of Women's Health*, that Native American postmenopausal women benefit from regular consumption of flaxseed by reducing their risk of cardiovascular disease, as observed by lowered LDL-C and TC levels. (24)

In 2008, the *British Journal of Nutrition* reported a study of the phytoestrogen properties of lignans derived from flaxseed. The treatments consisted of a placebo, 300 or 600 mg/day of dietary secoisolariciresinol diglucoside (SDG) from flaxseed extract. It was intended to determine the effect on plasma lipids and fasting glucose levels.

Significant treatment effects were achieved for the decrease of TC, LDL cholesterol (LDL-C) and glucose concentrations, as well as their percentage decrease from baseline. At weeks six and eight in the 600 mg SDG group, the decreases of TC and LDL-C concentrations were in the range of 22.0% to 24.38%, respectively compared to placebo. For the 300 mg SDG group, significant differences from baseline were observed only for decreases in TC and LDL-C.

Plasma glucose was found to be significantly lower in the 600 mg SDG group at weeks six and eight, especially in the participants with baseline glucose concentrations ≥ 5.83 mmol/l (lowered 25.56% and 24.96%) compared to placebo, respectively. Plasma concentrations of secoisolariciresinol (SECO), enterodiol (ED) and enterolactone were all significantly raised in the groups supplemented with flaxseed lignan. The observed cholesterol-lowering values were correlated with the concentrations of plasma SECO and ED. The investigators concluded that dietary flaxseed lignan extract decreased plasma cholesterol and glucose concentrations in a dose-dependent manner. (25)

A publication in the journal *Nutrition Reviews*, in 2004, was titled "Flaxseed and Cardiovascular risk." The investigators report that human studies have shown that flaxseed can reduce serum total and low-density lipoprotein cholesterol concentrations, reduce postprandial glucose absorption, decrease some markers of inflammation and raise serum levels of the omega-3 fatty acids, ALA and eicosapentaenoic acid. (26)

We know that the omega-3 fatty acids—especially ALA—in flaxseed and flax oil lower blood triglycerides (TC) and lipoproteins because omega-3 derived from other sources does it just as well. For instance:

A study published in the journal *Arteriosclerosis, Thrombosis and Vascular Biology* reported comparing the effect in volunteer participants of ingestion of 7 grams/day of omega-3, omega-6 or omega-9 fatty acids (EPA 41.4%, DHA 23.6%, providing a total of 4.55 grams of EPA/DHA) for four weeks versus no dietary intervention, on platelet-derived growth factor (PDGF-A, PDGF-B), heparin-bound epidermal growth factor (HB-EGF), monocyte chemoattractant protein-1 (MCP-1) and interleukin-10 gene expression in unstimulated Mononuclear Cells (MNCs) and in monocytes that were adherence-activated *ex vivo*.

These benefits were not found with omega-6 or omega-9 fatty acids. This demonstrates that omega-3 fatty acids can modulate inflammatory gene expression. MCP-1 induces monocyte activation and attraction and both MCP-1 and PDGF are thought to promote atherosclerosis.

Omega-6 PUFA via corn oil (providing LA 50.1%, saturated fats 12.9%) tended to increase PDGF-A and MCP-1 (although not significantly). (27)

PDGF is a platelet-derived growth factor. PDGFs are molecules released from platelets. Forms of PDGF help to heal wounds and to repair damage to blood vessel walls. They also help blood vessels grow.

In 2021, the journal *Current Problems in Cardiology* reported a systematic review and meta-analysis titled "Effects of Flaxseed on Blood Lipids in Healthy and Dyslipidemic Subjects." The study aimed to determine the effects of flaxseed on lipid profile in healthy and dyslipidemic individuals. The literature search was performed based on English reports of randomized control trials (RCTs) up to April 2021. It was found that flaxseed significantly improves the lipid profile in dyslipidemic patients comprising TC, LDL-C and triglyceride (TG) in comparison with the control group. In healthy individuals, flaxseed significantly increased HDL-C, LDL-C and TG.

Subgroup analysis on healthy subjects showed that flaxseed increased LDL-C on overweight subjects with BMI > 25. (28)

In a study published in the journal *Lancet*, patients awaiting carotid endarterectomy were given either sunflower oil (providing 3.6 grams of linoleic acid), fish oil or control until surgery with a median duration of treatment being 42 days. Compared to control and sunflower oil, EPA/DHA decreased the prevalence of thin fibrous caps, increased thick fibrous caps, reduced signs of inflammation and reduced the number of macrophages within plaques.

The investigators concluded that atherosclerotic plaques readily incorporate omega-3 PUFAs from fish oil supplementation, inducing changes that can enhance stability of atherosclerotic plaques. By contrast, increased consumption of omega-6 PUFAs does not affect carotid plaque fatty-acid composition or stability. (29)

Interestingly, it was also found in the aforementioned study that there were more thin fibrous cap atheromas (29.6% vs. 22.8%), fewer thick fibrous cap atheromas (53.7% vs. 56.1%) and a greater percentage of plaque rupture (5.6% vs. 3.5%) in the sunflower oil group vs. control, respectively. Although none of these differences were significant the numerical trend for worse plaque morphology with the intake of omega-6 PUFAs is concerning. Additionally, what is generally considered stable plaque tended to be lower in the sunflower group compared to the control group.

These clinical studies illustrate the benefits of omega-3 fatty acids, but they did not derive them from flaxseed or flax oil.

5.1.5 Omega-3 Fatty Acids from Flaxseed Lower Triglycerides

Triglycerides are composed of glycerol and three fatty acids. They are the main constituent of body fat. They are present in blood and enable the bidirectional transfer of adipose fat and blood glucose from the liver. In most people who do not have a genetic predisposition to hypertriglyceridemia, it is commonly associated with obesity, type 2 diabetes and metabolic syndrome.

While the clinical emphasis is usually on cholesterol, recent evidence suggests that triglyceride levels above normal raise risk of catastrophic cardiovascular disease. Here are the clinical ranges for triglycerides:

Clinical ranges of triglyceride levels (51)

Normal less than	150*
Borderline high	150–199
High	200–499
Very high	500 or higher

*All values in milligrams per deciliter.

In 2003, the *American Journal of Clinical Nutrition* reported that *"Dietary linolenic acid is inversely associated with plasma triacylglycerol"* as part of the National Heart, Lung, and Blood Institute, which showed that dietary ALA (highest quintile 1.24 grams/day) is associated with lower plasma triglycerides (TG) concentrations. (30)

5.1.6 L-Arginine (Abundant in Flaxseed) Prevents, Even Reverses, Atherosclerosis

L-arginine, a semi-essential α-amino acid, part of the biosynthesis of proteins, is naturally found in red meat, poultry, fish, dairy, beans and nuts and seeds. It is a precursor of NO essential to blood vessel and heart function, to brain and nervous system function and to immune system function. Each of these functions has its own dedicated form (isoforms) of catalyst synthase enzyme. These enzymes convert L-arginine to citrulline, producing NO in the process. Oxygen and NADPH are necessary cofactors.

A number of authorities hold that atherosclerosis is basically due to endothelial dysfunction. For instance, investigators writing in the *Journal of Molecular and Cellular Medicine* in 1999, conclude,

> *Endothelial dysfunction by aging, menopause and hypercholesterolemia is involved in the development of atherosclerotic vascular lesions, and predisposes the blood vessel to several vascular disorders, such as vasospasm and thrombosis. Multiple mechanisms are apparently involved in the pathogenesis of the endothelial dysfunction in atherosclerosis. The reduced production of nitric oxide by the endothelium is caused by abnormalities in endothelial signal transduction, availability of L-arginine, cofactors for endothelial nitric oxide synthase and expression of the enzyme. Other mechanisms may also be involved in the impaired endothelium-dependent relaxations in atherosclerosis, including increased destruction of nitric oxide by superoxide anion, altered responsiveness of vascular smooth muscle, and concomitant release of vasocontracting factors.* (31) With permission.

Even more directly, the author of a 1998 report in the *Journal of Investigative Medicine* titled his publication "Is Atherosclerosis an Arginine Deficiency Disease?" To wit, *"A reduction in NO synthesis and/or activity may contribute to the initiation and progressive of atherosclerosis. Derangement of the NO synthase pathway may occur by several mechanisms, including lipoproptein-induced alterations in signal transduction; increases in superoxide anion elaboration (and degradation of NO); reduced affinity of NOS for L-arginine; and/or elevated levels of circulating antagonists."* (32)

The "reduced affinity of NOS for L-arginine" is unlikely due to what is known as the *arginine paradox*: Exogenous L-arginine causes NO-mediated biological effects even when nitric oxide synthases (NOS) are saturated with L-arginine. (33) None of this is to discount the role of nutrition, oxidative stress and lifestyle factors that lead to the endothelial dysfunction associated with atherosclerosis.

A good number of studies have supported supplementing L-arginine orally or by infusion to control plaque formation. For instance, authors of a clinical study published in 1997 in the journal *Atherosclerosis* titled their report "Oral

L-Arginine Improves Endothelium-Dependent Dilatation and Reduces Monocyte Adhesion to Endothelial Cells in Young Men with Coronary Artery Disease." In this study, men with angiographically proven coronary atherosclerosis took 7 grams of L-arginine three times per day, or placebo, for three days with a ten-day wash-out period.

Following L-arginine, plasma levels of arginine rose significantly (318 ± 18 vs. 124 ± 9 mumol/l), and endothelium-dependent dilatation of the brachial artery measured as the change in diameter in response to reactive hyperaemia (FMD) using external vascular ultrasound improved significantly (4.7 ± 1.1 vs. 1.8 ± 0.7%). No such results were found in the placebo comparison. Serum from participants after L-arginine and placebo was then added to confluent monolayers of human umbilical vein endothelial cells for 24 hours before human monocytes obtained by countercurrent centrifugal elutriation (34) were added and cell adhesion assessed by light microscopy.

> *Centrifugal elutriation is a liquid clarification technique that makes it possible to separate different cells with different sizes. Since cell size is correlated with cell cycle stages this method also allows the separation of cells at different stages of the cell cycle.*

Adhesion was found to be significantly reduced following L-arginine compared to placebo (42 ± 2 vs. 50 ± 1%). The investigators, therefore, concluded that in young men with coronary artery disease, oral L-arginine improves endothelium-dependent dilatation and reduces monocyte/endothelial cell adhesion. (35)

In connection with the *arginine paradox*, the authors of a report published in the *Journal of Nutrition* in 2004 contend that the mechanism of benefit of L-arginine on endothelial function is unclear because intracellular concentrations of L-arginine far exceed that required by eNOS. One potential explanation of this "arginine paradox" is that L-arginine restores endothelial function in atherosclerotic patients in whom there are elevated levels of ADMA, an endogenous inhibitor of eNOS. (36)

A study conducted in Iran, published in 2014 in the journal *F1000 Research* aimed to evaluate the effect of low-dose L-arginine supplementation on cardiovascular disease (CVD) risk factors, including lipid profile, blood sugar and blood pressure in healthy Iranian men. For 45 days, the intervention group received 2,000 mg daily L-arginine supplementation. The control group received 2,000 mg of maltodextrin placebo daily.

At the end of study, fasting blood sugar and lipid profile, i.e, triglyceride (TG), cholesterol, LDL, HDL, decreased significantly in the L-arginine group but no significant change in the placebo group were found. In addition, reductions in fasting blood sugar and the lipid profile were significantly better than the control group. However, no significant changes were found in systolic and diastolic blood pressure either in L-arginine or placebo group. (37)

There are many more clinical and experimental (animal model) studies that could be cited to show the benefits of L-arginine of relevance to flaxseed or flax oil–derived L-arginine in lowering or even in reversing atherosclerosis. These studies go to the effect of enhancing eNO. As noted earlier, omega-3 enhances endothelial function and L-arginine is the substrate for NO. Likewise, cyanogenic glycosides (CNglcs) in flaxseed are NO-donors–flax oil, which is extracted from the seeds does not contain appreciable amounts of cyanogenic glycosides. No creditable studies of CNglcs from any source concerning atherosclerosis could be found.

5.2 CHRONIC SYSTEMIC INFLAMMATION

Chronic systemic inflammation (CSI) is also referred to as slow, long-term inflammation lasting for prolonged periods of several months to years. It results from the release of proinflammatory cytokines from immune-related cells and the chronic activation of the innate immune system. Diseases in which inflammation plays a dominant pathological role have the suffix "-itis."

Inflammation comes in two forms—acute and chronic. Acute inflammation helps us with the healing process and is generally short-lived. In chronic inflammation, the effects linger. Over time, chronic inflammation will have an adverse effect on tissues and organs. CSI plays a role in the development of many diseases ranging from autoimmune diseases to cancer.

Typical signs of CSI include fatigue, fever and joint and muscle pain. There are also atypical symptoms, including balance issues, insulin resistance, muscle weakness, eye problems, skin issues and more. More recently, atherosclerosis has been added to the list.

A report in the journal *Current Pharmaceutical Design* appearing in 2012 contends that

> atherosclerosis starts with an innate immune response involving the recruitment and activation of monocytes macrophages that respond to an excessive accumulation of modified lipids within the arterial wall, followed by an adaptive immune response involving antigen-specific T lymphocytes. Effector T cells recognize modified autoantigens such as oxidized LDL and heat shock proteins (i.e. HSP-60) that are presented by antigen-presenting cells such as macrophages or dendritic cells. The accumulation of inflammatory cells within the arterial wall leads to local production of chemokines, interleukins and proteases that enhance the influx of monocytes and lymphocytes, thereby promoting the progression of atherosclerotic lesions. (38)

The study was titled "Atherosclerosis as an Inflammatory Disease."

What is CSI? Is it a disease? Is it a *process* leading to disease? It is likely that it is both. In any case, the evidence for CSI is in the test known as C-reactive protein (CRP).

5.2.1 C-REACTIVE PROTEIN IN INFLAMMATION

C-Reactive protein (CRP) is an acute-phase protein of liver origin found in plasma that increases following interleukin-6 secretion by macrophages and T cells. Its circulating concentrations rise in response to inflammation. CRP is usually measured in milligrams of CRP per liter of blood (mg/L). Normal CRP levels are typically below 3.0 mg/L. But, the normal reference range often varies between labs.

The range of CRP in milligrams per liter of blood in adults and their clinical significance are as follows (52):

- Below 3.0: Normal
- 3.0–10.0: Slightly elevated, which may signify a variety of conditions, such as pregnancy, the common cold or gingivitis
- 10.0–100.0: Moderately elevated, which signifies infection or an inflammatory condition such as rheumatoid arthritis, Crohn's disease or lupus
- 100.0–500.0: Severely elevated, which signifies severe bacterial infection

A high-sensitivity CRP (hs-CRP) test can detect levels below 10.0 mg/L. This kind of test is performed primarily to determine a person's risk for heart disease. hs-CRP ranges in milligrams per liter of blood and heart disease risk (52):

- Below 1.0: Low risk
- 1.0–3.0: Moderate risk
- 3.0–10.0: High risk

CRP, an acute inflammatory protein that increases up to 1,000-fold at sites of infection or inflammation, is synthesized primarily in liver hepatocytes but also by smooth muscle cells, macrophages, endothelial cells, lymphocytes and adipocytes. (39) Some reports find CRP useful in evaluating the benefits of flaxseed and flax oil as an outcome measure in flaxseed or flax oil supplementation, while others find it limited to specific clinical populations. For instance:

In a meta-analysis titled "Effect of Flaxseed Intervention on Inflammatory Marker C-Reactive Protein," published in the journal *Nutrients* in 2016, the investigators reported that flaxseed and its derivatives may have a beneficial effect on reducing circulating CRP only in obese populations. (40)

The aim of a multicenter trial reported in the journal *Nutrition Research*, in 2012, was to determine the effects of flaxseed oil on inflammation in patients with chronic renal failure undergoing renal replacement therapy with hemodialysis (HD). It was hypothesized that flax oil supplementation would lower CRP levels. Patients received three dialysis sessions per week over a three-month period. They were given blind doses of 1 gram flax oil twice a day, and the control group was given 1 gram mineral oil placebo twice a day for a period of 120 days.

Inflammation was observed in 89 patients (61%) at the beginning of the study. There was a significant linear correlation between CRP and the body mass index and HDL cholesterol, and the CRP levels decreased significantly over time in the group that received flax oil compared to the control group. During the study period, 33.3% of the flax oil group no longer had inflammation whereas only 16.9% changed in the mineral oil group. The investigators concluded that flax oil decreases the CRP levels and that inflammation in hemodialysis patients appears to be correlated to their body mass index and reduced HDL cholesterol levels. (41)

In one clinical study (42), the intake of an ALA-rich diet of 6.5% of energy/day from ALA has led to a large 75% decrease in CRP levels in blood samples from hypercholesterolemic men and women. ALA appears to decrease CVD risk by inhibiting vascular inflammation and endothelial activation beyond its lipid-lowering effects.

In another independent study, ALA levels in a plasma cholesterol fraction have also been negatively correlated with CRP concentrations. In this study on overweight adolescents, published in the *American Journal of Clinical Nutrition* in 2005, eicosapentaenoic acid in phospholipids and cholesterol esters (CEs) and linolenic acid in CEs were significantly inversely related to CRP. These findings remained significant after adjustment for the waist-to-hip ratio. No significant relation between fatty acids composition and the homeostasis model assessment was observed.

The investigators concluded that a high intake of long-chain PUFAs, especially omega-3 PUFAs may protect obese subjects against metabolic syndrome and low-grade inflammation as early as adolescence. (43)

In yet another study published in the journal *Nutrition, Metabolism and Cardiovascular Diseases* in 2008, it was reported that secoisolariciresinol diglucoside (SDG) isolated from flaxseed (500 mg/day) reduced CRP concentration by approximately 15% in healthy postmenopausal women when they were compared with a placebo group during a six-week intervention period. (44)

We should be careful not to be misled by the results of studies that report no change in CRP consequent on flaxseed or flax oil supplementation because there may have been other clinically significant changes. However, it should be noted that there are publications that report no detectable change in CRP as a consequence of flax seed or flax oil supplementation. (45)

5.2.2 Omega-3 ALA Reduces Inflammation

A study published in the *Journal of Nutrition* in 2004 aimed to determine whether ALA could reduce the risk of CVD by lowering vascular inflammation and endothelial dysfunction. Inflammatory markers and lipids and lipoproteins were assessed in hypercholesterolemic participants fed two diets low in saturated fat and cholesterol and high in PUFAs varying in ALA (ALA Diet) and linoleic acid (LA Diet—omega-6), compared with an average American diet (AAD). The ALA Diet provided 17% energy from PUFA (10.5% LA; 6.5% ALA), the LA Diet provided 16.4% energy from PUFA (12.6% LA; 3.6% ALA) and the AAD provided 8.7% energy from PUFA (7.7% LA; 0.8% ALA).

The ALA diet significantly decreased CRP, whereas the LA Diet only *tended* to decrease CRP. Although the two high-PUFA diets similarly significantly decreased intercellular cell adhesion molecule-1 vs. AAD (−19.1% by the ALA Diet; −11.0% by the LA Diet), the ALA Diet significantly decreased vascular cell adhesion molecule-1 (VCAM-1, −15.6% vs. −3.1% and E-selectin (−14.6% vs. −8.1%) more than the LA Diet.

E-Selectin is a glycoprotein only expressed on endothelial cells after activation by interleukin 1 (IL-1), tumor necrosis factor α (TNFα), or bacterial lipopolysaccharides. Regulation of E-selectin expression might be crucial to control leukocyte accumulation in inflammatory responses. (50)

Changes in CRP and VCAM-1 were inversely associated with significant changes in serum eicosapentaenoic acid (EPA), or EPA plus docosahexaenoic (DHA) after subjects consumed the ALA Diet. The two high-PUFA diets significantly decreased serum total cholesterol, LDL cholesterol and triglycerides; the ALA Diet significantly decreased HDL cholesterol and apolipoprotein AI compared with the AAD. The investigators concluded that ALA appears to decrease CVD risk by inhibiting vascular inflammation and endothelial activation beyond its lipid-lowering effects. (42)

5.2.3 L-Arginine, *per se*, and Inflammation

An experimental study published in the *International Journal of Molecular Sciences* in 2019 reported that L-arginine exerts anti-inflammatory and antioxidant effects to protect IPEC-J2 cells from an inflammatory response and oxidative stress challenged by lipopolysaccharide at least partly via the Arg-1 signaling pathway. (46)

> - *IPEC-J2 cells are intestinal porcine enterocytes isolated from the jejunum of a neonatal unsuckled piglet.*
> - *The Arg-1 gene instructs the production of the enzyme arginase that participates in the urea cycle, a series of reactions that occurs in liver cells. The urea cycle processes excess nitrogen, which is generated when proteins and their building blocks (amino acids) are used by the body.*

We remind you that flaxseeds are abundant in arginine.

A review and meta-analysis of clinical studies titled "Effect of L-arginine Supplementation on C-Reactive Protein and Other Inflammatory Biomarkers" published in the journal *Complementary Therapies in Medicine* in 2019 concluded that L-arginine supplementation increased the circulating concentrations of CRP in individuals older than 60, in those with higher levels of CRP, in patients with cancer and when used in enteral formula. (47)

5.2.4 Flax/Omega-3 and Rheumatoid Arthritis

Rheumatoid arthritis is a chronic inflammatory autoimmune disorder that can affect joints, the skin, eyes, lungs, heart and blood vessels. Unlike osteoarthritis, it affects the lining of joints, causing a painful swelling that can eventually result in bone erosion, joint deformity and damage to other parts of the body as well. Signs and symptoms may include the following:

- Tender, warm, swollen joints
- Joint stiffness that is usually worse in the mornings and after inactivity
- Fatigue, fever and loss of appetite
- Early rheumatoid arthritis tends to affect smaller joints first—particularly the joints that attach the fingers to the hands and the toes to the feet

- As the disease progresses, symptoms often spread to the wrists, knees, ankles, elbows, hips and shoulders. In most cases, symptoms occur in the same joints on both sides of the body

Signs and symptoms may vary in severity and may even come and go. Periods of increased disease activity, called flares, alternate with periods of relative remission when the swelling and pain fade or disappear. Over time, rheumatoid arthritis can cause joints to deform and shift out of place.

A comprehensive literature search and meta-analysis published in the journal *Advances in Nutrition* in 2019 showed significant effects of flaxseed intake on circulating high-sensitivity CRP (hs-CRP) and TNFα. However, no significant changes were found in IL-6 concentration and CRP. Moreover, by eliminating one of the studies from the sensitivity analysis, changes in IL-6 concentration were significant. The changes in inflammatory biomarkers were dependent on study design (parallel or crossover), supplement type (flaxseed, flaxseed oil, or lignan), study quality (high or low) and participants' age and body mass index (BMI).

According to this meta-analysis, flaxseed significantly reduced circulating concentrations of hs-CRP and TNFα, but did not affect IL-6 and CRP. (48)

There is a report in the *American Journal of Clinical Nutrition* in 2000 that supplementation of omega-3 fatty acids has been consistently shown to reduce both the number of tender joints on physical examination and the amount of morning stiffness in patients with rheumatoid arthritis. In these cases, supplements were consumed daily in addition to background medications and the clinical benefits of the omega-3 fatty acids were not apparent until they were consumed for ≥ 12 wk.

A minimum daily dose of 3 grams of eicosapentaenoic and docosahexaenoic acids is necessary to derive the expected benefits. These doses of omega-3 fatty acids are associated with significant reductions in the release of leukotriene B(4) from stimulated neutrophils and of interleukin 1 from monocytes. Both of these mediators of inflammation are thought to contribute to the inflammatory events that occur in the rheumatoid arthritis disease process.

There have been a number of reports that rheumatoid arthritis patients consuming omega-3 dietary supplements were able to lower or discontinue their background doses of nonsteroidal anti-inflammatory drugs or disease-modifying anti-rheumatic drugs. However, the investigators contend that because the methods used to determine whether patients taking omega-3 supplements can discontinue taking these agents are variable, confirming and definitive studies are needed to settle this issue.

Omega-3 fatty acids have virtually no reported serious toxicity in the dose range used in rheumatoid arthritis and are generally very well tolerated. (49)

5.3 SUMMARY

Atherosclerosis and chronic systemic inflammation are grouped in this chapter because they are related, i.e., atherosclerosis is an inflammatory disease that begins with free radical oxidation of cholesterol. Studies have shown that both atherosclerosis and chronic systemic inflammation respond to flaxseed and flax oil supplementation because flax supplies both omega-3 fatty acids and L-arginine, the substrate for nitric oxide formation. Both are antioxidants and both support endothelium health.

5.4 REFERENCES

1. Bentzon JF, Otsuka F, Virmani R, and E Falk. 2014. Mechanisms of plaque formation and rupture. *Circulation Research*, Jun 6; 114(12): 1852–1866. DOI:10.1161/CIRCRESAHA.114.302721.
2. Wang JC, and M Bennett. 2012. Aging and atherosclerosis. Mechanisms, functional consequences, and potential therapeutics for cellular senescence. *Circulation Research*, Jul 6; 111(2): 245–259. DOI:10.1161/CIRCRESAHA.111.261388.
3. www.earthslab.com/physiology/vasa-vasorum/; accessed 11/5/21.
4. Ritman EL, and A Lerman. 2007. The dynamic vasa vasorum. *Cardiovascular Research*, Sep 1; 75(4): 649–658. DOI:10.1016/j.cardiores.2007.06.020.
5. Senoner T, and W Dichtl. 2019. Oxidative stress in cardiovascular diseases: Still a therapeutic target? *Nutrients*, Sep; 11(9): 2090. DOI:10.3390/nu11092090.
6. Staprans I, Pan X-M, Rapp JH, and KR Feingold. 2005. The role of dietary oxidized cholesterol and oxidized fatty acids in the development of atherosclerosis. *Molecular Nutrition and Food Research*, Nov; 49(11): 1075–1082. DOI:10.1002/mnfr.200500063.
7. Prasad K. 1997. Dietary flax seed in prevention of hypercholesterolemic atherosclerosis. *Atherosclerosis*, Jul 11; 132(1): 69–76. DOI:10.1016/s0021-9150(97)06110-8.8.
8. Francis AA, Deniset JF, Austria JA, and RK Lavallee. 2013. The effects of dietary flaxseed on atherosclerotic plaque regression. *American Journal of Physiology. Heart and Circulatory Physiology*, Jun 15; 304(12): H1743–H1751. DOI:10.1152/ajpheart.00606.2012.
9. Francis AA, Deniset JF, Austria JA, LaValleé RK, Maddaford GG, Hedley TE, Dibrov E, and GN Pierce. 2013. Effects of dietary flaxseed on atherosclerotic plaque regression. *American Journal of Physiology. Heart and Circulatory Physiology*, Jun 15; 304(12): H1743–1751. DOI:10.1152/ajpheart.00606.2012.
10. Zernecke A, Shagdarsuren E, and C Weber. 2008. Chemokines in atherosclerosis: An update. *Arteriosclerosis, Thrombosis and Vascular Biology*, Nov; 28(11): 1897–1908. DOI:10.1161/ATVBAHA.107.161174.
11. Johnson RC, Leopold JA, and J Loscalzo. 2009. Vascular calcification: Pathobiological mechanisms and clinical implications. *Circulation Research*, Sep 11; 105(6): e8. DOI:10.1161/01.RES.0000249379.55535.21.
12. Nowak WN, Deng J, Xiong Z, Ruan XZ, and Q Xu. 2017. Reactive oxygen species generation and atherosclerosis. *Arteriosclerosis, Thrombosis, and Vascular Biology*, May 1; 37(5): e41–e52. DOI:10.1161/ATVBAHA.117.309228.
13. Burtenshaw D, Hakimjavadi R, Redmond EM, and PA Cahill. 2017. Nox, reactive oxygen species and regulation of vascular cell fate. *Antioxidants* (Basel), Nov 14; 6(4): 90. DOI:10.3390/antiox6040090.
14. Burtenshaw D, Kitching M, Redmond EM, Megson IL, and PA Cahill. 2019. Reactive oxygen species (ROS), intimal thickening, and subclinical atherosclerotic disease. *Frontiers in Cardiovascular Medicine*, 6: 89. DOI:10.3389/fcvm.2019.00089.
15. Simopoulos AP. 2000. Human requirement for N-3 polyunsaturated fatty acids. *Poultry Science*, Jul; 79(7): 961–970. DOI:10.1093/ps/79.7.961.
16. Francois CA, Connor SL, Bolewicz LC, and WE Connor. 2003. Supplementing lactating women with flaxseed oil does not increase docosahexaenoic acid in their milk. *American Journal of Clinical Nutrition*, Jan; 77(1): 226–233. DOI:10.1093/ajcn/77.1.226.

17. Austria JA, Richard MN, Chahine MN, Edel AL, Malcolmson LJ, Dupasquier CMC, and GN Pierce. 2008. Bioavailability of alpha-linolenic acid in subjects after ingestion of three different forms of flaxseed. *Journal of the American College of Nutrition*, Apr; 27(2): 214–221. DOI:10.1080/07315724.2008.10719693.
18. Kuijsten A, Arts ICW, van't Veer P, and PCH Hollman. 2005. The relative bioavailability of enterolignans in humans is enhanced by milling and crushing of flaxseed. *Journal of Nutrition*, Dec; 135(12): 2812–2816. DOI:10.1093/jn/135.12.2812.
19. Arterburn LM, Bailey Hall EB, and H Oken. 2006. Distribution, interconversion, and dose response of n-3 fatty acids in humans. *American Journal of Clinical Nutrition*, Jun; 83(6 Suppl): 1467S–1476S. DOI:10.1093/ajcn/83.6.1467S.
20. Ghafoorunissa IM. 1992. N-3 fatty acids in Indian diets—comparison of the effects of precursor (alpha-linolenic acid) vs product (long-chain n-3 polyunsaturated fatty acids). *Nutrition Research*, 12: 569–582.
21. Patenaude A, Rodriguez-Leyva D, Edel AL, Dibrov E, Dupasquier CMC, Austria JA, Richard MN, Chahine MN, Malcolmson LJ, and GN Pierce. 2009. Bioavailability of alpha-linolenic acid from flaxseed diets as a function of the age of the subject. *European Journal of Clinical Nutrition*, Sep; 63(9): 1123–1129. DOI:10.1038/ejcn.2009.41.
22. Thiébaut ACM, Chajès V, Gerber M, Boutron-Ruaul M-C, Joulin V, Lenoir G, Berrino F, Riboli E, Bénichou J, and F Clavel-Chapelon. 2009. Dietary intakes of omega-6 and omega-3 polyunsaturated fatty acids and the risk of breast cancer. *International Journal of Cancer*, Feb 15; 124(4): 924–931. DOI:10.1002/ijc.23980.
23. Nestel PJ, Pomeroy SE, Sasahara T, Yamashita T, Liang YL, Dart AM, Jennings GL, Abbey M, and JD Cameron. 1997. Arterial compliance in obese subjects is improved with dietary plant n-3 fatty acid from flaxseed oil despite increased LDL oxidizability. *Arteriosclerosis, Thrombosis and Vascular Biology*, Jun; 17(6): 1163–1170. DOI:10.1161/01.atv.17.6.1163.
24. Patade A, Devareddy L, Lucas EA, Korlagunta K, Daggy BP, and BH Arjmandi. 2008. Flaxseed reduces total and LDL cholesterol concentrations in Native American postmenopausal women. *Journal of Women's Health* (Larchmt), Apr; 17(3): 355–366. DOI:10.1089/jwh.2007.0359.
25. Zhang W, Wang X, Liu Y, Tian H, Flickinger B, Empie MW, and SZ Sun. 2008. Dietary flaxseed lignan extract lowers plasma cholesterol and glucose concentrations in hypercholesterolaemic subjects. *British Journal of Nutrition*, Jun; 99(6): 1301–1309. DOI:10.1017/S0007114507871649.
26. Bloedon LeA T, and PO Szapary. 2004. Flaxseed and cardiovascular risk. *Nutrition Reviews*, Jan; 62(1): 18–27. DOI:10.1111/j.1753-4887.2004.tb00002.x.
27. Baumann KH, Hessel F, Larass I, Müller T, Angerer P, Kiefl R, and C von Schacky. 1999. Dietary omega-3, omega-6, and omega-9 unsaturated fatty acids and growth factor and cytokine gene expression in unstimulated and stimulated monocytes. A randomized volunteer study. *Arteriosclerosis, Thrombosis, and Vascular Biology*, Jan; 19(1): 59–66. DOI:10.1161/01.atv.19.1.59.
28. Masjedi MS, Pour PM, Yalda Shokoohinia Y, and S Asgary. 2021. Effects of flaxseed on blood lipids in healthy and dyslipidemic subjects: A systematic review and meta-analysis of randomized controlled trials. *Current Problems in Cardiology*, Available online 16 July 2021. https://doi.org/10.1016/j.cpcardiol.2021.100931.
29. Thies F, Garry JMC, Yaqoob P, Rerkasem K, Shearman CP, Gallagher PJ, Calder PC, and RF Grimble. 2003. Association of n-3 polyunsaturated fatty acids with stability of atherosclerotic plaques: A randomised controlled trial. *Lancet*, Feb 8; 361(9356): 477–485. DOI:10.1016/S0140-6736(03)12468-3.
30. Djoussé L, Hunt SC, Arnett DK, Province MA, Eckfeldt JH, and RC Ellison. 2003. Dietary linolenic acid is inversely associated with plasma triacylglycerol: The National

Heart, Lung, and Blood Institute family heart study. *American Journal of Clinical Nutrition*, Dec; 78(6): 1098–1102. DOI:10.1093/ajcn/78.6.1098.
31. Shimokawa HJ. 1999. Primary endothelial dysfunction: Atherosclerosis. *Journal of Molecular and Cellular Medicine*, Jan; 31(1): 23–37. DOI:10.1006/jmcc.1998.0841.
32. Cooke JP. 1998. Is atherosclerosis an arginine deficiency disease? *Journal of Investigative Medicine*, Oct; 46(8): 377–380. PMID: 9805422.
33. Nakaki T, and K Hishikawa. 2002. The arginine paradox. *Nihon Yakurigaku zasshi. Folia Pharmacologica Japonica*, Jan 1; 119(1): 7–14. DOI:10.1254/fpj.119.
34. Banfalvi G. 2008. Cell cycle synchronization of animal cells and nuclei by centrifugal elutriation. *Nature Protocols*, Mar; 3(4): 663–673. DOI:10.1038/nprot.2008.34.
35. Adams MR, McCredie R, Jessup W, Robinson J, Sullivan D, and DS Celermajer. 1997. Oral L-arginine improves endothelium-dependent dilatation and reduces monocyte adhesion to endothelial cells in young men with coronary artery disease. *Atherosclerosis*, Mar 21; 129(2): 261–269. DOI:10.1016/s0021-9150(96)06044-3.
36. Gornik HL, and MA Creager. 2004. Arginine and endothelial and vascular health. *Journal of Nutrition*, Oct; 134(10 Suppl): 2880S–2887S; discussion 2895S. DOI:10.1093/jn/134.10.2880S.
37. Pahlavani N, Jafari M, Sadeghi O, Rezaei M, Rasad H, Rahdar HA, and MH Entezaria. 2014. L-Arginine supplementation and risk factors of cardiovascular diseases in healthy men: A double-blind randomized clinical trial. *F1000 Research*, Dec; 3: 306. DOI:10.12688/f1000research.5877.2.
38. Tuttolomondo A, Di Raimondo D, Pecoraro R, Arnao V, Pinto A, and G Licata. 2012. Atherosclerosis as an inflammatory disease. *Current Pharmaceutical Design*, 18(28): 4266–4288. DOI:10.2174/138161212802481237.
39. Sproston NR, and JJ Ashworth. 2018. Role of C-reactive protein at sites of inflammation and infection. *Frontiers in Immunology*, Apr 13; 9: 754. DOI:10.3389/fimmu.2018.00754.
40. Ren GY, Chen CY, Chen GC, Chen WG, Pan A, Pan CW, Zhang YH, Qin LQ, and LH Chen. 2016. Effect of flaxseed intervention on inflammatory marker C-Reactive Protein: A systematic review and meta-analysis of randomized controlled trials. *Nutrients*, Mar 4; 8(3): 136. DOI:10.3390/nu8030136.
41. Lemos JRN, Gascue de Alencastro M, Vieceli Konrath AV, Cargnin M, and RC Manfro. 2012. Flaxseed oil supplementation decreases C-reactive protein levels in chronic hemodialysis patients. *Nutrition Research*, Dec; 32(12): 921–927. DOI:10.1016/j.nutres.2012.08.007.
42. Zhao G, Etherton TD, Martin KR, West SG, Gillies PJ, and PM Kris-Etherton. 2004. Dietary alpha-linolenic acid reduces inflammatory and lipid cardiovascular risk factors in hypercholesterolemic men and women. *Journal of Nutrition*, Nov; 134(11): 2991–2997. DOI:10.1093/jn/134.11.2991.
43. Klein-Platat C, Drai J, Oujaa M, Schlienger J-L, and C Simon. 2005. Plasma fatty acid composition is associated with the metabolic syndrome and low-grade inflammation in overweight adolescents. *American Journal of Clinical Nutrition*, Dec; 82(6): 1178–1184. DOI:10.1093/ajcn/82.6.1178.
44. Hallund J, Tetens I, Bügel S, Tholstrup T, and JM Bruun. 2008. The effect of a lignan complex isolated from flaxseed on inflammation markers in healthy postmenopausal women. *Nutrition, Metabolism and Cardiovascular Diseases*, Sep; 18(7): 497–502. DOI:10.1016/j.numecd.2007.05.007.
45. Ursoniu S, Sahebkar A, Serban M-C, Pinzaru I, Dehelean C, Noveanu L, Rysz J, and M Banach. 2019. Lipid and Blood Pressure Meta-analysis Collaboration (LBPMC) group. *Archives of Medical Sciences*, Jan; 15(1): 12–22. DOI:10.5114/aoms.2018.81034.

46. Qiu Y, Yang X, Wang L, Gao K, and Z Jiang. 2019. L-Arginine inhibited inflammatory response and oxidative stress induced by lipopolysaccharide via arginase-1 signaling in IPEC-J2 cells. *International Journal of Molecular Sciences*, Apr; 20(7): 1800. DOI:10.3390/ijms20071800.
47. Nazarian B, Moghadam EF, Asbaghi O, Khosroshahi MZ, Choghakhori R, and A Abbasnezhad. 2019. Effect of l-arginine supplementation on C-reactive protein and other inflammatory biomarkers: A systematic review and meta-analysis of randomized controlled trials. *Complementary Therapies in Medicine*, Dec; 47: 102226. DOI:10.1016/j.ctim.2019.102226.
48. Rahimlou M, Jahromi NB, Hasanyani N, and AR Ahmadi1. 2019. Effects of flaxseed interventions on circulating inflammatory biomarkers: A systematic review and meta-analysis of randomized controlled trials. *Advances in Nutrition*, Nov; 10(6): 1108–1119. DOI:10.1093/advances/nmz048.
49. Kremer JM. 2000. n-3 fatty acid supplements in rheumatoid arthritis. *American Journal of Clinical Nutrition*, Jan; 71(1 Suppl): 349S–351S. DOI:10.1093/ajcn/71.1.349s.
50. Mantovani A, and E Dejana. 1998. Endothelium. In *Encyclopedia of immunology*, 2nd ed., MA: Academic Press/Elsevier. 802–806. https://doi.org/10.1006/rwei.1999.0212.
51. National Cholesterol Education Program. www.health.harvard.edu/heart-health/should-you-worry-about-high-triglycerides; accessed 11/7/21.
52. www.healthline.com/health/rheumatoid-arthritis-crp-levels#normal-crp-levels.

6 Flaxseed and L-Arginine, and Omega-3 Fatty Acids, *per se*, in Treatment of Hypertension and Sickle Cell Disease

6.1 HYPERTENSION

This chapter makes the case for flaxseed supplementation in controlling blood pressure and in treating sickle cell disease because its two main active constituents, L-arginine and omega-3 fatty acid, have demonstrated clinical effectiveness.

In 2017, the American College of Cardiology and the American Heart Association (AHA) published new guidelines for hypertension management and defined hypertension as having blood pressure at or above 130/80 mm Hg. Hypertension raises the risk of heart disease, stroke, peripheral vascular disease, kidney disease and many more medical disorders, which are leading causes of death in the United States. In 2019, more than half a million deaths in the United States had hypertension as a primary or contributing cause. (1) It cost the United States about $131 billion each year, averaged over 12 years from 2003 to 2014.

Hypertension is largely a "silent" disease, but there are sometimes symptoms such as the following:

- Severe headaches
- Nosebleeds
- Fatigue or confusion
- Vision problems
- Chest pain
- Difficulty breathing
- Irregular heartbeat
- Blood in the urine

It is often first detected during a routine periodic medical checkup.

Common factors that can lead to high blood pressure are said to be a diet high in salt, fat and/or cholesterol and a sedentary lifestyle. It is a primary risk factor for cardiovascular disease, including stroke, heart attack, heart failure, kidney failure and aneurysm. Keeping blood pressure under control is vital for preserving health

6.1.1 HYPERTENSION AS OMEGA-3 DEFICIENCY

In a previous chapter, it was reported that atherosclerosis might be an L-arginine deficiency disease. (2) "Deficiency" does not necessarily mean "lack of" in the conventional sense, especially in light of the *arginine paradox* that the nitric oxide synthase (NOS) enzyme is often supersaturated. It might just mean that something interferes with or prevents its normal function, i.e., perhaps a dysfunctional or missing enzyme or cofactor. We raise this issue here because a number of authorities make the parallel suggestion that hypertension may, in many cases, be an omega-3 deficiency disease. There is considerable scientific support for this notion.

We will revisit the question, "Could hypertension be a deficiency disease?" in any sense, later in this chapter—see ADMA.

But to the point, it was shown in an experimental animal-model study (Sprague–Dawley rats) that omega-3 polyunsaturated fatty acid deficiency, particularly during the prenatal period, can cause hypertension in later life. (3) Additionally, when deficiency is reversed in later life, omega-3 fatty acid levels are essentially restored while hypertension remains. (4) The issue is further confounded by the fact that, as reported in the journal *Hypertension* in 2010, body fat and leptin may be factors involved in omega-3 fatty acid deficiency hypertension. (5)

Maternal deprivation of omega-3 fatty acids has been shown to result in (animal) infants that develop hypertension. Dietary omega-3 fatty acid deficiency can lead to hypertension in later life. We can lower blood pressure in adults with hypertension with omega-3. But what is the effect of altering the dietary protein level on blood pressure in animals deficient or sufficient in omega-3 fatty acids?

In an experimental study reported in the *American Journal of Hypertension* in 2010, female rats were placed on one of four experimental diets one week prior to mating. Diets were either deficient (10% safflower oil; DEF) or sufficient (7% safflower oil, 3% flaxseed oil; SUF) in omega-3 fatty acids and contained 20% or 30% casein (DEF20, SUF20, DEF30, SUF30). Offspring were maintained on the maternal diet for the duration of the experiment. At 12, 18, 24 and 30 weeks, blood pressure was assessed by tail-cuff plethysmography.

It was found that at both 12 and 18 weeks of age, no differences in blood pressure were observed based on diet. However, by 24 weeks, hypertension was evident in DEF30 animals; there were no significant blood pressure differences between the other groups. This hypertension in DEF30 group was increased at 30 weeks, with systolic, diastolic and mean arterial pressure all significantly elevated.

The investigators concluded that the hypertension previously attributed to omega-3 fatty acid deficiency is also dependent on additional dietary factors, including protein content of the diet. (6)

There is evidence also, as reported in the journal *BMJ* in 2003, that prenatal omega-3 fatty acid supplementation may reduce diastolic blood pressure in human infants as well. (7) It is consistent with these findings that the Mediterranean Diet, rich in omega-3, may be thought to help reduce blood pressure.

The Greek Mediterranean Diet prior to the 1960s provided adequate consumption of the essential omega-3 fatty acids with the ratio omega-3/omega-6 of 2:1. (8) This, parenthetically, is in contrast to the current diet of Greeks with the total omega- 6 to omega-3 ratio of about 10:1, which is closer to the Western Diet of 15:1.

This increase in the ratio is unfortunate because, as reported in a study published in the *Journal of the American College of Nutrition* in 2001, omega-6 fatty acids, and especially linoleic acid (AL), in disproportionate amounts, cause endothelial cell dysfunction most markedly as well, and it can potentiate TNF-mediated endothelial cell injury and is, therefore, atherogenic. (9)

Reporting in the journal *Current Vascular Pharmacology* in 2012, the investigators contend that there is considerable evidence that people with essential hypertension, i.e., high blood pressure that doesn't have a known primary cause, suffer endothelial dysfunction caused by impaired nitric oxide (NO) availability secondary to oxidative stress. (10, 11, 12) More about that next.

That given, there is also considerable evidence that flaxseed and flax oil lower blood pressure by their beneficial effect on endothelial health: Their omega-3 fatty acids are antioxidants, and both L-arginine and cyanogenic glycosides are NO-donors.

6.1.2 Flax/Omega-3 Fatty Acids Reduces Blood Pressure— The Harris Omega-3 Index

In a study published in the *Journal of Hypertension* in 2018, investigators hypothesized that the *Omega-3 Index* (defined next) would be inversely associated with blood pressure (BP) levels in young healthy adults. Participants with cardiovascular disease, known diabetes or a body mass index (BMI) higher than 35kg/m2 were excluded from the study. It was found that a higher Omega-3 Index is associated with statistically significant, clinically relevant lower systolic and diastolic blood pressure.

Based on the findings, the investigators recommended diets rich in omega-3 fatty acids for primary prevention of hypertension. (13)

> *The Omega-3 Index test is a measure of the amount of EPA and DHA in the blood, specifically in the red blood cell membranes. The Omega-3 Index test yields a percentage. For example, if there are 64 fatty acids in a cell membrane and three are EPA and DHA, then the Omega-3 Index is 4.6%.*

An Omega-3 Index of 8% or higher is ideal, the lowest risk zone. However, most American consumers are at 4% or less, the highest risk zone. Being in the highest risk zone translates to a 90% higher risk of sudden cardiac death. Here are the "risk zones" for coronary heart disease developed by Dr. WS Harris and colleagues, published in the *American Journal of Clinical Nutrition* in 2008 (14):

- Risk Zones: Omega-3 Index
- High Risk   = <4%

- Intermediate Risk = 4%–8%
- Low Risk   = >8%

The following study is particularly noteworthy because the authors conclude, "*In summary, flaxseed induced one of the most potent antihypertensive effects achieved by a dietary intervention.*" The clinical trial published in the journal *Hypertension* in 2013 aimed to determine the effects of daily flaxseed on systolic blood pressure (SBP) and diastolic blood pressure (DBP) in peripheral artery disease patients. Patients were given a variety of foods that contained 30 grams of milled flaxseed, or a placebo, each day for more than six months.

Plasma levels of the omega-3 fatty acid ALA and enterolignans rose significantly— 2- to 50-fold—in the flaxseed-fed group but did not increase significantly in the placebo group. SBP was ≈ 10 mm Hg lower, and DBP was ≈ 7 mm Hg lower in the flaxseed group compared with placebo after six months. Patients who entered the trial with a SBP ≥ 140 mm Hg at baseline saw a significant reduction of 15 mm Hg in SBP and 7 mm Hg in DBP from flaxseed consumption. The antihypertensive effect was achieved selectively in hypertensive patients: Circulating ALA levels correlated with SBP and DBP and lignan levels correlated with changes in DBP.

As noted earlier the investigators concluded that "flaxseed induced one of the most potent antihypertensive effects achieved by a dietary intervention." (15)

The purpose of the following review and meta-analysis, published in the *Journal of Nutrition* in 2015, was to determine the effect of flaxseed consumption on blood pressure and also the influence of baseline blood pressure, type of flaxseed supplementation and duration of flaxseed supplementation on blood pressure.

The analysis comprised PubMed (Medline), Cumulative Index to Nursing and Allied Health Literature and Cochrane Library (Central), through July 2014 for studies where people supplemented their habitual diet with flaxseed or its extracts (i.e., oil, lignans, fiber) for ≥2 weeks.

The investigators concluded that consumption of flaxseed may somewhat lower blood pressure, but the benefit is greater, especially for DBP, when it is consumed as a whole seed and for more than 12 weeks. (16)

A study reported in the *American Journal of Hypertension* in 2011 aimed to assess how modest variations in omega-3 fatty acid intake might affect blood pressure (BP) in a healthy community sample. The participants included Pittsburgh-area adults 30 to 54 years of age (11% black, 51% female) not taking omega-3 fatty acid supplements or antihypertensive medications. Standardized assessments of clinic and 24-hour ambulatory BP and pulse rate were obtained.

Docosahexanenoic acid (DHA) and eicosapentaenoic acid (EPA) in fasting serum phospholipids were measured. Analyses controlled for age, gender, race, BMI, self-reported sodium intake and physical activity.

It was found that DHA was inversely associated with clinic DBP, awake ambulatory DBP and 24-hour DBP. A significant increase in DHA was associated with 2.1 mm Hg lower in-clinic and 2.3 mm Hg lower awake ambulatory DBP. In addition, DHA was inversely associated with pulse rate measured at rest in the clinic.

The investigators concluded that in this sample of American adults not on antihypertensive medications, a modest albeit significant inverse association was found between DHA exposure and both clinic and ambulatory DBP. Therefore, increasing

DHA consumption through diet modification, rather than large dose supplementation, might be an effective strategy for preventing hypertension. (17)

While omega-3 fatty acids may have blood pressure (BP)–lowering effects in untreated hypertensive and elderly patients, their effect on BP in young, healthy adults remains unknown. A study published in the *Journal of Hypertension* in 2018, aimed to determine whether the omega-3 Index is inversely associated with BP in young healthy adults. The study investigated the baseline characteristics of a cohort that included healthy adults aged 25 to 41 years. Individuals with cardiovascular disease, known diabetes or a BMI higher than 35 kg/m were excluded.

It was found that median Omega-3 Index was 4.58%. Compared to individuals in the lowest Omega-3 Index quartile, individuals in the highest had a SBP and DBP that was significantly lower (4 and 2 mm Hg lower, respectively). A significant linear inverse relationship of the Omega-3 Index with 24-hour and office BP was observed. These findings are statistically significant. It was concluded that a higher Omega-3 Index is associated with statistically significant, clinically relevant lower SBP and DBP levels in normotensive young and healthy individuals. Furthermore, diets rich in omega-3 fatty acids may be a strategy for the primary prevention of hypertension. (13)

6.1.3 The Safety of Cyanogenic Glycosides in Flaxseed

One tablespoon of ground flaxseed weighs about 10 grams. It holds about 7 grams of fatty acids of which 1,800 mg is omega-3. One tablespoon of flax oil holds about 14,000 mg of omega 3. One tablespoon of ground flaxseed holds about 198 mg of L-arginine.

According to the Nutraceutical Alliance, regarding cyanogenic glycoside (CNglcs) in flaxseed, the main safety concern is with crushed or ground fresh flaxseed, not whole flaxseed from which little cyanide is formed and released when consumed, nor flax oil which is extracted from the seed and does not contain appreciable amounts of CNglcs nor the enzymes needed to produce cyanide from cyanogenic glycosides. The normal content of CNglcs precursors present in flaxseed from many sources in different continents ranges from less than 80 up to about 300 mg cyanide-equivalents/kg seed. (18)

Based on data from a study by Abraham, Buhrke and Lampen (2016), consuming 30 grams, ca. 3 tablespoons, of flaxseed with a cyanogenic precursor content of 200 mg/kg seed will result in an average peak blood cyanide concentration of 5 μmol/L. This is less than the toxic threshold value of 20 to 40 μmol/L favored by the European Food Safety Authority.

Using their data as a guide, as much as 120 grams of crushed/ground flaxseed can be consumed before a toxic threshold of 40 μmol/L is reached. Given that a tablespoon of ground flaxseed weighs about 10 grams, this amounts to about 12 tablespoons.

Cyanogenic glycosides are cited here in connection with the treatment of hypertension because, like L-arginine, they are NO-donors. But there are no studies in conventional journals that address CNglcs in that connection. There is, however, an intriguing review titled "Inflammation, Its Regulation and Antiphlogistic Effect of the CNglcs Amygdalin" (amygdalin, AKA cyanogenic glycoside), not drawn from flaxseed, that appeared in the journal *Molecules* in 2021. (19)

6.1.4 L-ARGININE SUPPLEMENTATION REDUCES BLOOD PRESSURE

Given that the NO-donor L-arginine supplements reduce blood pressure, it is reasonable to speculate that if that, therefore, flaxseed would logically reduce blood pressure since flaxseed contains available L-arginine. Therefore, we present data here on the benefits of L-arginine supplementation not necessarily obtained from flaxseed. This is due to the fact that clinical studies that cite flaxseed or flax oil *per se* in connection with blood pressure/hypertension typically do that on the basis of omega-3 content and, for unknown reasons, ignore the role of L-arginine. Here is what can be expected from L-arginine supplementation via flaxseed.

What actually happens in the body when L-arginine is administered either orally or by intravenous infusion? This question is answered by a clinical study published in the *British Journal of Clinical Pharmacology* in 1998 that addressed the "pharmacokinetic-pharmacodynamic relationship" in L-arginine-induced vasodilation in healthy people after a single intravenous infusion of 30 grams or 6 grams of L-arginine, or after a single oral application of 6 grams, as compared with the respective placebo. It was found that the vascular effects of L-arginine are closely correlated with its plasma concentrations.

The investigators contend that "these data may provide a basis for the utilization of L-arginine in cardiovascular diseases." (20)

The Western(ized) Diet is characterized by a high content of proteins mostly derived from fatty domesticated animals and processed meats. It stands to reason that such a diet should provide an ample supply of L-arginine. Indeed, it does, and L-arginine deficiency is therefore rare. Yet, as shown in the sample of clinical studies cited next, supplementing L-arginine has been shown in countless clinical reports to lower blood pressure. How can we explain this?

For openers, endothelium dysfunction comes to mind: A clinical study published in the *Journal of the American College of Cardiology* in 1992 titled "Abnormal Endothelium-Dependent Coronary Vasomotion in Hypertensive Patients" aimed to assess the integrity of endothelium-dependent vasodilation, the response of coronary arteries to acetylcholine (an endothelium-dependent vasodilator) and nitroglycerin (an endothelium-independent vasodilator) in patients undergoing cardiac catheterization.

Patients with essential hypertension were compared to normotensive patients. None had obstructive disease detectable by coronary arteriography. Coronary artery diameter was measured with digital-subtracted arteriography and coronary blood flow velocity with a Doppler flow velocity catheter. At baseline, coronary artery diameter was similar in the hypertensive and the normotensive control patients (2.4 ± 0.3 vs. 2.8 ± 0.7 mm).

During intracoronary acetylcholine infusion (30 micrograms/min), coronary artery diameter decreased significantly to 1.3 ± 0.7 mm in the hypertensive patients, but it was unchanged (2.7 ± 0.8 mm) in the normotensive patients. With intracoronary nitroglycerin (200 micrograms), coronary artery diameter increased significantly in both groups. Coronary blood flow decreased during acetylcholine infusion by $59 \pm 31\%$ in the hypertensive patients but increased by $3 \pm 3\%$ in the normotensive group. There was a significant negative correlation between the percent change in estimated coronary blood flow during acetylcholine infusion and mean arterial pressure measured at baseline.

Therefore, these hypertensive patients exhibited marked coronary vasoconstriction in response to intracoronary acetylcholine but normal vasodilation in response to nitroglycerin, suggesting abnormal endothelium-dependent vasodilation. (21)

Likewise, investigators reported a clinical study in the *New England Journal of Medicine* in 1990. They aimed to determine if patients with essential hypertension have an endothelium-dependent abnormality in vascular relaxation. They examined the response of the forearm vasculature to acetylcholine (an endothelium-dependent vasodilator) and sodium nitroprusside (a direct dilator of vascular smooth muscle) in hypertensive patients averaging 50.7 years of age (±10 years), two weeks after the withdrawal of antihypertensive medications.

The drugs were infused at increasing concentrations into the brachial artery and the response in forearm blood flow was measured by strain-gauge plethysmography. It was found that the basal forearm blood flow was similar in the patients and controls. The responses of blood flow and vascular resistance to acetylcholine were significantly reduced in the hypertensive patients. However, there were no significant differences between groups in the responses of blood flow and vascular resistance to sodium nitroprusside.

Because the effect of acetylcholine might also be due to presynaptic inhibition of the release of norepinephrine by adrenergic nerve terminals, it was assessed during phentolamine-induced, alpha-adrenergic blockade. Under these conditions, it was also evident that the responses to acetylcholine were significantly blunted in hypertensive patients. The investigators concluded that endothelium-mediated vasodilation is impaired in patients with essential hypertension. (22)

The authors of a review titled "The Antihypertensive Effect of Arginine," reported in the *International Journal of Angiology* in 2008, that the blood pressure-lowering effect of the Dietary Approaches to Stop Hypertension (DASH) study may be due to its higher arginine-containing protein, higher antioxidants (and low salt content). (23)

The aim of a review published in the journal *Nutrients* in 2019 was to determine whether oral administration of the amino acids L-arginine and L-citrulline, potential substrates for eNO, could effectively reduce blood pressure (BP) by increasing NO production. Both arginine and citrulline effectively increase plasma arginine.

The investigators report that oral arginine supplementation can lower BP by 5.39/2.66 mm Hg, which is an effect that is comparable to diet changes and exercise implementation.

They contend that the exact mechanism by which citrulline and arginine exert their effect is obscured because normal plasma arginine concentration greatly exceeds the Michaelis constant (K_m) of eNOS. Thus, elevated plasma arginine concentrations would not be expected to increase endogenous NO production significantly, but have nonetheless been observed to do so. This phenomenon reflects the "arginine paradox." (24)

The Michaelis(–Menten) equation characterizes the enzymatic rate at different substrate concentrations. (25)

A clinical study reported in the *International Journal of Cardiology* in 2002 conducted on patients with essential hypertension administered either 6 grams of L-arginine or a placebo. Patients were examined for flow-mediated, endothelium-dependent dilatation of the brachial artery (FMD) before and one-and-a-half hours after administration of L-arginine or placebo.

The two groups of L-arginine and placebo were similar regarding age, sex, blood lipids, smoking, diabetes, coronary artery disease, body mass index, intima-media thickness of the common carotid artery, clinics blood pressure and baseline brachial artery parameters. It was found that at the end of the trial, heart rate, blood pressure, baseline diameter, blood flow or reactive hyperemia did not change significantly. However, L-arginine resulted in a significant improvement of flow-mediated dilatation (FMD) while placebo did not significantly change this parameter. The effect of L-arginine on FMD was significantly different from the effect of placebo. L-Arginine did not significantly influence nitrate-induced dilatation.

It was concluded that oral administration of L-arginine acutely improves endothelium-dependent FMD of the brachial artery in patients with essential hypertension. (26)

The *Journal of Chiropractic Medicine* published an "umbrella review," i.e., a review of previously published systematic reviews or meta-analyses that encompassed the literature from January 1, 1980, through December 31, 2015, of three separate databases—PubMed, Cochrane Library and Cumulative Index to Nursing and Allied Health Literature.

The seven meta-analyses that were included in this umbrella review reported significant positive benefits of L-arginine on reducing systolic and DBP in hypertensive adults by 2.2 to 5.4 mm Hg and 2.7 to 3.1 mm Hg, respectively, reducing DBP in pregnant women with gestational hypertension by 4.9 mm Hg and reducing the length of stay in the hospital for surgical patients.

In addition, two of the three meta-analyses indicated a 40% reduction in the incidence of hospital-acquired infections. However, these positive results should be considered with caution because statistically significant heterogeneity was observed in five of the seven meta-analyses.

The investigator concluded that there is evidence to support the benefit of L-arginine supplementation for reducing systolic and diastolic blood pressure in hypertensive adults and reducing the incidence of hospital-acquired infections and the length of stay in the hospital for surgical patients. (27)

Simply put, the effectiveness of L-arginine in reducing blood pressure and controlling hypertension is not in doubt—it works. Here follow some additional interesting applications and findings: For instance, as reported in a clinical trial published in the journal *Chest* in 1996, healthy men were given a 30-minute infusion of 0.5 g/kg L-arginine hydrochloride. They underwent continuous monitoring of BP and heart rate (HR), as well as intermittent determination of mixed expired NO concentration and plasma L-arginine and L-citrulline levels. Infusion of L-arginine produced a significant fall in mean BP with a peak effect of $-9.3 \pm 0.9\%$.

The hemodynamic effects of L-arginine were associated with a significant increase in mixed *expired* NO concentration (FeNO) and a significant increase in the rate of pulmonary NO excretion of $118 \pm 45\%$, as well as a rise in plasma

L-citrulline from 25 ± 4 to 46 ± 5 μmol/L. There was a significant correlation between the hypotensive response to L-arginine and the increase in expired NO. According to the investigators, the hypotensive effect of L-arginine in humans appears to be mediated, at least in part, by NO synthase metabolism of L-arginine and increased endogenous NO production as indicated both by increased plasma L-citrulline and by increased expired NO. (28)

Based on these findings, it should be possible to use expired NO as an indirect measure of endothelium health. It is surprising that this is not routine because the technology for measuring expired NO has existed for some time now.

6.1.5 STUDIES CITING FLAXSEED OR FLAX OIL, PER SE, AND HYPERTENSION

Most studies of the effects of flaxseed or flax oil on blood pressure cite omega-3 as the active constituent. We found no clinical studies that actually cited flaxseed, per se, in treatment of hypertension.

6.1.6 COULD IT BE DUE TO ASYMMETRIC DIMETHYLARGININE (ADMA) WHEN L-ARGININE FAILS?

Asymmetric dimethylarginine (ADMA) is an analogue of L-arginine that is a naturally occurring product of metabolism found in human circulation. Elevated levels of ADMA inhibit NO formation, impairing endothelial function and thus promoting atherosclerosis. ADMA levels are increased in people with hypercholesterolemia, atherosclerosis, hypertension, chronic heart failure, diabetes mellitus and chronic renal failure. A number of studies have reported ADMA as a novel risk marker of cardiovascular disease.

Elevated levels of ADMA have been shown to be the strongest risk predictor, beyond traditional risk factors, of cardiovascular events and all-cause and cardiovascular mortality in people with coronary artery disease. Interventions such as treatment with L-arginine have been shown to improve endothelium-mediated vasodilatation in people with high ADMA levels. (29)

According to Mayo Clinic Laboratories also, ADMA is an independent risk factor for major adverse cardiovascular events. It inhibits NO synthesis and is elevated in diseases related to endothelial dysfunction, including hypertension, hyperlipidemia, and type 2 diabetes.

Elevation in ADMA and subsequent NO synthesis inhibition leads to vasoconstriction, reduced peripheral blood flow and reduced cardiac output. Baseline ADMA remained a significant risk factor for adverse, events even after adjusting for low-density lipoprotein cholesterol (LDL-C), high-density lipoprotein cholesterol (HDL-C), triglycerides, creatinine and high-sensitivity C-reactive protein. (39)

A number of studies, including one published in the journal *Current Cardiology Reviews* in 2010, have reported increased levels of ADMA to be the strongest risk predictor of cardiovascular events and all-cause and cardiovascular mortality in people with coronary artery disease. Interventions such as treatment with L-arginine have been shown to improve endothelium-mediated vasodilatation in people with high ADMA levels. (29)

The author of a report titled "Does ADMA Cause Endothelial Dysfunction?" published in the journal *Arteriosclerosis, Thrombosis, and Vascular Biology* in 2000 contends that

> Asymmetric dimethylarginine (ADMA) is an endogenous and competitive inhibitor of nitric oxide synthase. Plasma levels of this inhibitor are elevated in patients with atherosclerosis and in those with risk factors for atherosclerosis. In these patients, plasma ADMA levels are correlated with the severity of endothelial dysfunction and atherosclerosis. By inhibiting the production of nitric oxide, ADMA may impair blood flow, accelerate atherogenesis, and interfere with angiogenesis. ADMA may be a novel risk factor for vascular disease. (30) With permission.

In a review published in the journal *Alternative Medicine Review* in 2005, the authors concluded that the endothelium plays a crucial role in the maintenance of vascular tone and structure via endothelium-derived NO formed in healthy vascular endothelium from the amino acid L-arginine. Endothelial dysfunction is caused by cardiovascular risk factors, metabolic diseases and systemic or local inflammation. One possible cause of endothelial dysfunction is elevated blood levels of ADMA, an L-arginine analogue that inhibits NO formation and can, therefore, impair vascular function. Supplementation with L-arginine can restore vascular function and improve the clinical symptoms of diseases associated with vascular dysfunction. (31)

ADMA is of no small concern because, as noted earlier, it is a feature of hypertension but in addition, it is considered an extremely high risk of coronary catastrophe. (32)

6.1.6.1 Does ADMA Explain the Arginine Paradox?

We asked previously whether the *arginine paradox* could result from a malfunctioning or missing enzyme or cofactor. The author of a report in the *Journal of Nutrition* in 2004 proposes that elevated ADMA levels may explain the arginine paradox, i.e., the observation that supplementation with exogenous L-arginine improves NO-mediated vascular functions *in vivo*, although its baseline plasma concentration is about 25-fold higher than the Michaelis-Menten constant (Km) of the isolated, purified endothelial NO synthase *in vitro*.

According to the author, the biochemical and physiological pathways related to ADMA are well understood: Dimethylarginines are the result of degradation of methylated proteins. The methyl group is derived from S-adenosylmethionine. Both ADMA and its regioisomer, symmetric dimethylarginine, are eliminated from the body by renal excretion, whereas only ADMA is metabolized via hydrolytic degradation to citrulline and dimethylamine by the enzyme dimethylarginine dimethylaminohydrolase (DDAH). Decreases in DDAH activity and/or expression may therefore contribute to the pathogenesis of endothelial dysfunction in various diseases. Administration of L-arginine is suggested because it has been shown to improve endothelium-dependent vascular functions in subjects with high ADMA levels. (33)

Parenthetically, not only does L-arginine reduce levels of ADMA, but there is some evidence that polyunsaturated fatty acids (PUFAs) may do so also. But the evidence consists mainly of a small number of experimental animal studies. (34)

6.2 ENDOTHELIAL DYSFUNCTION IN SICKLE CELL DISEASE AND L-ARGININE THERAPY

Endothelial dysfunction is a known feature of sickle cell disease (SCD), which is present both in crisis and in steady state in children and adults with that disorder. Flaxseed delivers L-arginine, shown to be helpful in treatment of sickle cell disease because that disease is characterized by endothelium dysfunction, and L-arginine is a NO-donor. Flaxseed also delivers omega-3—alpha-linolenic acid and other PUFAs. Omega-3 has also been shown to be beneficial in connection with treatment of sickle cell disease.

The authors of a 2019 publication in the journal *Expert Review of Hematology* contend that,

> Considering the complex pathogenesis of the disease and the restricted access to curative therapies, the management of SCD must rely on a combination of therapies covering multiple pathways. Arginine supplementation, a low-cost approach, has shown promising results, which is particularly important considering most of the affected patients still live in unfavorable socioeconomic conditions. These findings should encourage further clinical trials, evaluating other outcomes and specific subpopulations, such as adult patients and compound heterozygotes. (35) With permission.

A study of Sudanese SCD patients, including children and adults aged 2 to 24 years, published in the *American Journal of Clinical Nutrition* in 2013, reported that omega-3 fatty acids significantly reduced the frequency of pain episodes from a median of 4.6 down to 2.7 per year, and of pain requiring hospitalization from a median of one down to zero per year. It also significantly reduced the frequency of severe anemia from 16.4% down to 3.2% per year and of transfusion from 16.4% down to 4.5% per year. (36)

It has been shown that endothelium dysfunction is a key feature of SCD. In a clinical study published in the journal, *Kidney 360*, investigators aimed to determine the relationship between endothelial dysfunction, biomarkers of renal dysfunction, and biomarkers of disease severity in asymptomatic SCD patients with renal disease.

Patients with homozygous SCD in steady state and age- and sex-matched controls were enrolled between 2013 and 2014 in a tropical tertiary hospital. Ultrasonographic FMD of the right brachial artery, renal arterial Doppler, complete blood count, creatinine, fetal hemoglobin, soluble P-selectin and cystatin C (Cys-C) levels were determined. Using the median FMD value of the control group, the SCD subjects were further classified into two groups for comparison.

It was found that the median FMD in SCD patients (3.44) was significantly lower than that of controls (5.35). There was a significant negative correlation between FMD and Cys-C levels, along with renal artery resistivity index in SCD patients. Additionally, Cys-C level was significantly higher in SCD subjects with FMD below 5.35.

The investigators concluded that brachial artery FMD is significantly lower in SCD patients compared to the control group, Cys-C and Renal Artery Resistance Index showing a negative correlation with FMD indicates that renal function is related to endothelial dysfunction in SCD. (37) Given that a key feature of SCD is endothelial dysfunction, L-arginine might play a role in reducing this aspect of the disease. In fact, that was shown in the following study:

The investigators of a clinical study published in the journal *Haematologica* in 2013 reiterate that low NO bioavailability contributes to vasculopathy in SCD. They hypothesized that arginine may be a beneficial treatment for pain related to SCD because L-arginine is the substrate for NO production, and an acute deficiency is associated with the pain of vaso-occlusive episodes.

Children with SCD hospitalized for at least 56 episodes of pain were enrolled in the study. They received 100 mg/kg tid of L-arginine or placebo for five days, or until they were discharged. As a result, there was a significant reduction in total parenteral opioid use of 54%, and lower pain scores at discharge were reported in the treatment group, compared to the placebo group. There was no significant difference in the length of stay in the hospital, although a trend favored the arginine group.

The investigators concluded that arginine therapy represents a novel intervention for painful vaso-occlusive episodes because it resulted in a "remarkable" reduction of narcotic use by more than 50%. (38)

Surprisingly, no studies on the effects of flax, *per se*, in the treatment of SCD could be found.

6.3 SUMMARY

Clinical as well as experimental (animal) studies have shown that endothelium dysfunction and impaired bioavailability of NO are both principal features of hypertension and SCD. Flaxseed delivers L-arginine and CNglcs, both NO-donors, to lower blood pressure and to relieve pain episodes in sickling. In addition, it delivers omega-3 fatty acid shown to improve endothelium dysfunction underlying both conditions. Although evidence of clinical flaxseed administration, *per se*, in hypertension and in SCD is limited, many studies confirm the beneficial effects of L-arginine and omega-3 fatty acids, *per se*, in treatment of these medical conditions.

6.4 REFERENCES

1. No authors listed. 2019. Centers for Disease Control and Prevention, National Center for Health Statistics. *About multiple cause of death, 1999–2019.* CDC WONDER Online Database website. Atlanta, GA: Centers for Disease Control and Prevention.
2. Cooke JP. 1998. Is atherosclerosis an arginine deficiency disease? *Journal of Investigative Medicine*, Oct; 46(8): 377–380. PMID: 9805422.
3. Armitage JA, Pearce AD, Sinclair AJ, Vingrys AJ, Weisinger RS, and HS Weisinger. 2003. Increased blood pressure later in life may be associated with perinatal n-3 fatty acid deficiency. *Lipids*, Apr; 38(4): 459–464. DOI:10.1007/s11745-003-1084-y.
4. Weisinger HS, Armitage JA, Sinclair AJ, Vingrys AJ, Burns PL, and RS Weisinger. 2001. Perinatal omega-3 fatty acid deficiency affects blood pressure later in life. *Nature Medicine*, Mar; 7: 258–259. DOI:10.1038/85354.
5. Begg DP, Sinclair AJ, Stahl LA, Premaratna SD, Hafandi A, Jois M, and RS Weisinger. 2010. Hypertension induced by ω-3 polyunsaturated fatty acid deficiency is alleviated by α-linolenic acid regardless of dietary source. *Hypertension Research*, Mar; 7: 258–259. DOI:10.1038/hr.2010.84.

6. Begg DP, Sinclair AJ, Stahl LA, Garg ML, Jois M, and RS Weisinger. 2010. Dietary protein level interacts with omega-3 polyunsaturated fatty acid deficiency to induce hypertension. *American Journal of Hypertension*, Feb; 23(2): 125–128. DOI:10.1038/ajh.2009.198.
7. Forsyth JS, Willatts P, Agostoni C, Bissenden J, Casaer P, and G Boehm. 2003. Long-chain polyunsaturated fatty acid supplementation in infant formula and blood pressure in later childhood: Follow up of a randomised controlled trial. *BMJ*, May 3; 326(7396): 953. DOI:10.1136/bmj.326.7396.953.
8. Anagiotakos DB, Kastorini C-M, Pitsavos C, and C Stefanadis. 2011. The current Greek diet and the omega-6/omega-3 balance: The Mediterranean Diet score is inversely associated with the omega-6/omega-3 ratio. In: Simopoulos AP, ed. *Healthy Agriculture, Healthy Nutrition, Healthy People*. World Review of Nutrition and Dietetics. Basel: Karger, vol. 102, pp. 53–56. DOI:10.1159/000327791.
9. Hennig B, Toborek M, and CJ McClain. 2001. High-energy diets, fatty acids and endothelial cell function: Implications for atherosclerosis. *Journal of the American College of Nutrition*, Apr; 20(2 Suppl): 97–105. DOI:10.1080/07315724.2001.10719021.
10. Ghiadon L, Taddei S, and A Virdis 2012. Hypertension and endothelial dysfunction: Therapeutic approach. *Current Vascular Pharmacology*, 10: 42–60. DOI:10.2174/157016112798829823.
11. Savoia C, Sada L, Zezza L, Pucci L, Lauri FM, Befani A, Alonzo A, and M Volpe. 2011. Vascular inflammation and endothelial dysfunction in experimental hypertension. *International Journal of Hypertension*, Sep 11; 2011: 281240. DOI:10.4061/2011/281240.
12. Dharmashankar K, and ME Widlansky. 2010. Vascular endothelial function and hypertension: Insights and directions. *Current Hypertension Reports*, 12: 448–455. DOI:10.1007/s11906-010-0150-2.
13. Filipovic MG, Aeschbacher S, Reiner MF, Stivala S, Gobbato S, Bonetti N, Risch M, Risch L, Camici GG, Luescher TF, von Schacky C, Conen D, and JH Beera. 2018. Whole blood omega-3 fatty acid concentrations are inversely associated with blood pressure in young, healthy adults. *Journal of Hypertension*, Jul; 36(7): 1548–1554. DOI:10.1097/HJH.0000000000001728.
14. Harris WS. 2008. The omega-3 index as a risk factor for coronary heart disease. *American Journal of Clinical Nutrition*, Jun; 87(6): 1997S–2002S. DOI:10.1093/ajcn/87.6.1997S.
15. Rodriguez-Leyva D, Weighell W, Edel AL, LaVallee R, Dibrov E, Pinneker R, Maddaford TG, Ramjiawan B, Aliani M, Guzman R, and GN Pierce. 2013. Potent antihypertensive action of dietary flaxseed in hypertensive patients. *Hypertension*, Dec; 62(6): 1081–1089. DOI:10.1161/hypertensionaha.113.02094.
16. Khalesi S, Irwin C, and M Schubert. 2015. Flaxseed consumption may reduce blood pressure: A systematic review and meta-analysis of controlled trials. *Journal of Nutrition*, Apr; 145(4): 758–765. DOI:10.3945/jn.114.205302.
17. Liu JC, Conklin SM, Manuck SB, Yao JK, and MF Muldoon. 2011. Long-chain omega-3 fatty acids and blood pressure. *American Journal of Hypertension*, Oct; 24(10): 1121–1126. DOI:10.1038/ajh.2011.120.
18. Abraham K, Buhrke T, and A Lampen. 2016. Bioavailability of cyanide after consumption of a single meal of foods containing high levels of cyanogenic glycosides: A crossover study in humans. *Archives of Toxicology*, 90(3): 559–574. DOI:10.1007/s00204-015-1479-8.
19. Figurová D, Tokárová K, Greifová H, Knížatová N, Kolesárová A, and N Lukáč. 2021. Inflammation, it's regulation and antiphlogistic effect of the cyanogenic glycoside amygdalin. *Molecules*, Oct; 26(19): 5972. DOI:10.3390/molecules26195972.
20. Bode-Böger SM, Böger RH, Galland A, Tsikas D, and JC Frölich. 1998. L-Arginine-induced vasodilation in healthy humans: Pharmacokinetic-pharmacodynamic relationship. *British*

Journal of Clinical Pharmacology, Nov; 46(5): 489–497. DOI:10.1046/j.1365-2125. 1998.00803.x.
21. Brush JE Jr, Faxon DP, Salmon S, Jacobs AK, and TJ Ryan. 1992. Abnormal endothelium-dependent coronary vasomotion in hypertensive patients. *Journal of the American College of Cardiology*, Mar 15; 19(4): 809–815. DOI:10.1016/0735-1097(92)90522-o.
22. Panza JA, Quyyumi AA, Brush JE Jr, and SE Epstein. 1990. Abnormal endothelium-dependent vascular relaxation in patients with essential hypertension. *New England Journal of Medicine*, Jul 5; 323(1): 22–27. DOI:10.1056/NEJM199007053230105.
23. Vasdev S, and V Gill. 2008. The antihypertensive effect of arginine. *International Journal of Angiology*, Spring; 17(1): 7–22. DOI:10.1055/s-0031-1278274.
24. Khalaf D, Krüger M, Wehland M, Infanger M, and D Grimm. 2019. The effects of oal l-Arginine and L-citrulline supplementation on blood pressure. *Nutrients*, Jul; 11(7): 1679. DOI:10.3390/nu11071679.
25. Michaelis L, and ML Menten. 1913. Die Kinetik der Invertinwirkung. *Biochemische Zeitschrift*, 49: 333–369.
26. Lekakis JP, Papathanassiou S, Papaioannou TG, Papamichael CM, Zakopoulos N, Kotsis V, Dagre AG, Stamatelopoulos K, Protogerou A, and SF Stamatelopoulos. 2002. Oral L-arginine improves endothelial dysfunction in patients with essential hypertension. *International Journal of Cardiology*, Dec; 86(2–3): 317–323. DOI:10.1016/s0167-5273(02)00413-8.
27. McRae MP. 2016. Therapeutic benefits of l-Arginine: An umbrella review of meta-analyses. *Journal of Chiropractic Medicine*, Sep; 15(3): 184–189. DOI:10.1016/j.jcm.2016.06.002.
28. Mehta S, Stewart DJ, and RD Levy. 1996. The hypotensive effect of L-arginine is associated with increased expired nitric oxide in humans. *Chest*, Jun; 109(6): 1550–1555. DOI:10.1378/chest.109.6.1550.
29. Sibal L, Agarwal SC, Home PD, and RH Boger. 2010. The Role of asymmetric dimethylarginine (ADMA) in endothelial dysfunction and cardiovascular disease. *Current Cardiology Reviews*, May; 6(2): 82–90. DOI:10.2174/157340310791162659.
30. Cooke JP. 2000. Does ADMA cause endothelial dysfunction? *Arteriosclerosis, Thrombosis, and Vascular Biology*, Sep; 20(9): 2032–2037. DOI:10.1161/01.atv.20.9.2032.
31. Böger RH, and ES Ron. 2005. L-Arginine improves vascular function by overcoming deleterious effects of ADMA, a novel cardiovascular risk factor. *Alternative Medicine Review*, Mar; 10(1): 14–23. PMID: 15771559.
32. Valkonen VK, Paiva H, Laaksonen R, Lakka TA, Lehtimäki T, Laakso J, and R Laaksonen. 2001. Risk of acute coronary events and serum concentration of asymmetrical dimethyl arginine. *Lancet*, Dec 22; 358(9299): 2127–2130. DOI:10.1016/S0140-6736(01)07184-7.
33. Böger RH. 2004. Asymmetric dimethylarginine, an endogenous inhibitor of nitric oxide synthase, explains the "L-arginine paradox" and acts as a novel cardiovascular risk factor. *Journal of Nutrition*, Oct; 134(10 Suppl): 2842S–2847S. DOI:10.1093/jn/134.10.2842S.
34. Raimondi L, Lodovici M, Visioli F, Sartiani L, Cioni L, Alfarano C, Banchelli G, Pirisino R, Cecchi E, Cerbai E, and A Mugelli. 2005. n-3 polyunsaturated fatty acids supplementation decreases asymmetric dimethyl arginine and arachidonate accumulation in aging spontaneously hypertensive rats. *European Journal of Nutrition*, Sep; 44(6): 327–333. DOI:10.1007/s00394-004-0528-5.
35. Benites BD, and ST Olalla-Saad. 2019. An update on arginine in sickle cell disease. *Expert Review of Hematology*, Apr; 12(4): 235–244. DOI:10.1080/17474086.2019.1591948.
36. Daak AA, Ghebremeskel K, Hassan Z, Attallah B, Azan HH, Elbashir MI, and M Crawford. 2013. Effect of omega-3 (n-3) fatty acid supplementation in patients with sickle

cell anemia: Randomized, double-blind, placebo-controlled trial. *American Journal of Clinical Nutrition*, Jan; 97(1): 37–44. DOI:10.3945/ajcn.112.036319.
37. Ayoola OO, Bolarinwa RA, Onwuka CC, Idowu BM, and AS Aderibigbe. 2020. Association between endothelial dysfunction, biomarkers of renal function, and disease severity in sickle cell disease. *Kidney 360*, Feb; 1 (2): 79–85. DOI:10.34067/KID.0000142019.
38. Morris CR, Kuyper FA, Lavrisha L, Ansari M, Sweeters N, Stewar M, Gildengorin G, Neumayr L, and EP. Vichinsky. 2013. A randomized, placebo-controlled trial of arginine therapy for the treatment of children with sickle cell disease hospitalized with vaso-occlusive pain episodes. *Haematologica*, Sep; 98(9): 1375–1382. DOI:10.3324/haematol.2013.086637.
39. Mayo Clinic Laboratories: No authors listed. No date listed. www.mayocliniclabs.com/test-catalog/Clinical+and+Interpretive/607697; accessed 11/18/21.

7 L-Arginine and Omega-3 Fatty Acids in Adjuvant Treatment for Type 2 Diabetes and Chronic Kidney Disease

7.1 THE CONTRIBUTION OF FLAXSEED CONSTITUENTS IN TYPE 2 DIABETES MELLITUS

Research and clinical studies label treatments based on flaxseed in accordance with what, in the flaxseed, is thought to be the principal dependent variable. It could be "flaxseed," *per se*, or its omega-3 polyunsaturated fatty acids (PUFAs). However, it is almost never L-arginine and never CNglcs that are proposed as the active agent. For that reason, this chapter details the treatment of type 2 diabetes and chronic kidney disease (CKD) with L-arginine separate and apart from the omega-3 PUFAs because supplementing or adjuvant treatment with flaxseed must, of necessity, include the ample L-arginine contained in flaxseeds.

Both L-arginine and omega-3 fatty acids have shown success in clinical trials in the adjuvant treatment of type 2 diabetes and in kidney failure when they were administered separately. Cyanogenic glycosides (CNglcs) in flaxseed are also NO-donors like L-arginine. However, their specific contribution to diabetes and kidney disease can only be surmised because there is no published clinical trial evidence. It is reasonable to assume, however, that the contribution of CNglcs is imbedded in the outcome of flaxseed *per se* supplementation trials and in L-arginine from flaxseed trials.

Type 2 diabetes is characterized by high levels of glucose in the blood. It is a chronic impairment in the regulation of blood glucose caused either by insulin resistance, where cells respond poorly to it, or where the pancreas does not produce sufficient insulin. More than 34 million Americans have diabetes (about 1 in 10), and approximately 90% to 95% have type 2 diabetes. Most often, type 2 diabetes develops in people over age 45, but more and more children, teens and young adults are developing it.

Type 2 diabetes is an expanding global health problem closely linked to the epidemic of obesity. Individuals with type 2 diabetes are at high risk for both microvascular complications including retinopathy, nephropathy and neuropathy, and micro- and macrovascular complications such as cardiovascular comorbidities due to hyperglycemia and individual components of the insulin resistance metabolic syndrome.

Environmental factors, obesity, an unhealthy diet, physical inactivity and genetic factors contribute to the multiple pathophysiological disturbances that are responsible for impaired glucose homeostasis in type 2 diabetes. But insulin resistance and impaired insulin secretion remain the core defects. (1)

While deranged glucose metabolism is certainly a *prima facie* feature of type 2 diabetes, the problems that the condition causes relate to the effects of reactive oxygen species (ROS) it generates *en masse* and the resulting oxidative stress. Therefore, the two features of type 2 diabetes that concern us are inflammation and the resulting endothelial dysfunction that leads to the well-known consequences of that disease.

7.1.1 Oxidative Stress in Type 2 Diabetes

There are numerous reports of the damaging role played by ROS in diabetes in studies showing that oxygen radical damage greatly increases in type 2 diabetes and that this condition is often characterized by abnormalities in antioxidant defenses.

For instance, the aim of a study published in the journal *Acta Medica* in 2005 was to determine whether there is a relationship between the severity of type 2 diabetes retinopathy and leukocyte superoxide dismutase (SOD), catalase (CAT) activities and lipid peroxidation (LPO). Leukocyte malondialdehyde (MDA) levels, SOD and CAT activities were measured in patients with type 2 diabetes mellitus and nondiabetic healthy control participants.

- Superoxide dismutase(s) SODs form the front line of defense against ROS-mediated injury.
- Catalase enzyme brings about (catalyzes) the reaction by which hydrogen peroxide is decomposed to water and oxygen.

It was found that LPO, a natural component of the immune system, in the type 2 diabetic patients with retinopathy was significantly higher, whereas SOD and CAT activities were significantly lower compared to those of controls. MDA concentrations (see the following) rose, while SOD and CAT activities fell with increasing severity of diabetic retinopathy.

The investigators concluded that leukocytes in patients with type 2 diabetic retinopathy are affected by oxidative stress, which might contribute to the pathogenesis of the retinopathy. (2)

> *Free radicals generate lipid peroxidation. MDA is one of the final products of PUFA peroxidation in the cells. An increase in free radicals causes overproduction of MDA. MDA level is commonly known as a marker of oxidative stress and antioxidant status. (3)*

Just as oxidative stress is considered to be a damaging factor in type 2 diabetes so too can antioxidants neutralize it. This was shown in a clinical study published in the journal *Diabetes Care* in 2004. The aim of the study was to determine whether antioxidant intake could predict type 2 diabetes. The study centered on a cohort of men and women 40 to 69 years of age, free of diabetes at baseline. Food consumption during the previous year was estimated using a dietary history interview, and intake of vitamin C, four tocopherols, four tocotrienols and six carotenoids were determined. Follow-up lasted 23 years.

It was found that vitamin E intake was significantly associated with a reduced risk of type 2 diabetes. Intakes of α-tocopherol, γ-tocopherol, δ-tocopherol and β-tocotrienol were inversely related to a risk of type 2 diabetes. Among single carotenoids, β-cryptoxanthin intake was significantly associated with a reduced risk of type 2 diabetes. The investigators concluded that development of type 2 diabetes may be reduced by the intake of antioxidants in the diet. (4)

Some prospective studies have shown that higher vegetable and fruit consumption may lower the risk of developing diabetes, suggesting that antioxidants in the diet may have a synergistic effect. For instance, a study published in *Diabetes Care* in 1995 investigated the role of diet as a predictor of glucose intolerance and type 2 diabetes.

At the 30-year follow-up survey of the Dutch and Finnish cohorts of the Seven Countries Study (1989/1990), men were examined according to a standardized protocol, including a two-hour oral glucose tolerance test. Information on habitual food consumption was obtained using the *cross-check dietary history* method, (5) a dietary survey method to estimate the habitual food consumption of individuals. Those men in whom information on habitual diet was also available 20 years earlier were included in this study. Participants with known diabetes in 1989/1990 were excluded from the analyses.

It was found that adjusting for age and cohort, the intake of total saturated and monounsaturated fatty acids and dietary cholesterol 20 years before diagnosis was higher in men with newly diagnosed diabetes in the survey than in men with normal or impaired glucose tolerance. After adjustment for cohort, age, past body mass index and past energy intake, the past intake of total fat was significantly positively associated with two-hour, post-load glucose level. There was a significant inverse association with the past intake of vitamin C. These associations were independent of changes in the intake of fat and vitamin C during the 20-year follow-up. A greater consumption of vegetables and legumes, potatoes and fish during the 20-year follow-up was found to be significantly inversely related to two-hour glucose level.

The investigators concluded that these results indicate that a high intake of fat, especially that of saturated fatty acids, contributes to the risk of glucose intolerance and type 2 diabetes, while foods such as fish, potatoes, vegetables and legumes may have a protective effect. Furthermore, the observed inverse association of vitamin C and glucose intolerance suggests that antioxidants may also play a role in the development of derangements in glucose metabolism. (6)

A prospective study watches for outcomes, such as the development of a disease, during the study period and relates this to other factors, such as suspected risk.

7.1.2 ENDOTHELIAL DYSFUNCTION IN TYPE 2 DIABETES

Having shown in the previous section that ROS plays an adverse role in type 2 diabetes, it remains now to show that its adverse impact is on the endothelium. Endothelial dysfunction has received increasing attention as a potential contributor to the pathogenesis of vascular disease in diabetes mellitus: the delicate balanced release of endothelial-derived relaxing and contracting factors is altered in diabetes, thereby contributing to further progression of vascular and end-organ damage. (7)

A clinical study published in the *Journal of the American Medical Association* in 2004 aimed to assess the relationship between the biomarkers of endothelial dysfunction and the risk of type 2 diabetes. Elevated plasma levels of biomarkers reflecting endothelial dysfunction (E-selectin; intercellular adhesion molecule 1 [ICAM-1]; and vascular cell adhesion molecule 1 [VCAM-1]) were shown to predict development of type 2 diabetes in initially nondiabetic women.

In a prospective study within the Nurses' Health Study, an ongoing US study initiated in 1976, women who were initially enrolled provided blood samples from 1989 to 1990. Controls were selected according to matching age, fasting status and race.

It was found that baseline median levels of the biomarkers E-selectin, 61.2 vs. 45.4 ng/mL; ICAM-1, 264.9 vs. 247.0 ng/mL; and VCAM-1, 545.4 vs. 526.0 ng/mL were significantly higher among type 2 diabetes cases than among controls. Elevated E-selectin and ICAM-1 levels predicted incident diabetes. The adjusted relative risks for incident diabetes in the top quintile vs. the bottom quintiles were 5.43 for E-selectin, 3.56 for ICAM-1 and 1.12 for VCAM-1.

> *E-selectin (CD62E) is a glycoprotein expressed on endothelial cells only after activation by interleukin 1 (IL-1), tumor necrosis factor α (TNFα) or bacterial lipopolysaccharides. E-selectin expression might be crucial to controlling leukocyte accumulation in inflammatory responses. ICAM-1 plays a role in inflammatory processes and in the T-cell mediated host defense system. VCAM-1 protein mediates the adhesion of lymphocytes, monocytes, eosinophils and basophils to vascular endothelium. It also functions in leukocyte-endothelial cell signal transduction, and it may play a role in the development of atherosclerosis and rheumatoid arthritis.*

Adjustment for waist circumference instead of body mass index (BMI) or further adjustment for baseline levels of C-reactive protein (CRP), fasting insulin and hemoglobin Hba1c or exclusion of cases diagnosed during the first four years of follow-up did not alter these findings.

The investigators concluded that endothelial dysfunction predicts type 2 diabetes in women independent of other known risk factors, including obesity and subclinical inflammation. (8) Given these findings, one might reasonably expect that flaxseed taken as a whole, because it contains antioxidant omega-3 fatty acids as well as the NO-donor L-arginine (and the NO-donor cyanogenic glycosides), should have a significant beneficial effect on type 2 diabetes.

7.2 FLAXSEED AS ADJUVANT TREATMENT OF TYPE 2 DIABETES

A number of functional foods have been shown to possess hypoglycemic properties. (9) Flaxseed is a functional food that is rich in omega-3 fatty acids and other antioxidants and is low in carbohydrates. Flaxseed contains 32% to 45% of its mass as oil of which 51% to 55% is *alpha*-linolenic acid (ALA).

Research titled "In Vivo and In Vitro Antidiabetic and Anti-Inflammatory Properties of Flax (*Linum usitatissimum* L.) Seed Polyphenols," published in a report in the journal *Nutrients* in 2021, was conducted on mice and Wistar rats. It found 18 active polyphenols and concluded that they may serve as dietary supplements or novel phytomedicines to treat diabetes and its complications. (10)

A clinical *open-label* study on the effect of flax seed powder in the management of diabetes—a trial where participants and investigators know which treatment/substance each one is receiving—was published in the *Journal of Dietary Supplements* in 2011. The study aimed to determine the efficacy of flaxseed supplementation in type 2 diabetes.

The experimental group diet was supplemented daily with 10 grams of flaxseed powder for a period of one month. The control group received no supplementation or placebo. During the study, diet and drug regimen of the participants were unaltered. The efficacy of supplementation with flaxseed was evaluated by a battery of clinico-biochemical parameters.

Supplementation with flaxseed significantly reduced fasting blood glucose by 19.7% and glycated hemoglobin (HbA1c) by 15.6%. A favorable significant reduction in total cholesterol (14.3%), triglycerides (17.5%), low-density lipoprotein cholesterol (21.8%), apolipoprotein B and a significant increase in high-density lipoprotein cholesterol (11.9%) were also noticed.

These observations suggest the therapeutic potential of flaxseed in the management of diabetes mellitus. (11) There are in addition, many randomized blind-control studies, reviews and meta-analyses with positive outcome reports. For example:

A clinical study published in the journal *Nutrition Research* in 2013 aimed to determine whether, in overweight or obese individuals with pre-diabetes, fasting glucose, insulin, fructosamine, CRP, interleukin-6 will decrease and adiponectin will increase with daily flaxseed consumption.

> *Serum fructosamine is a glycated protein.*

Overweight or obese men and postmenopausal women with pre-diabetes consumed 0.0, 13 or 26 grams of ground flaxseed for 12 weeks. Glucose, insulin, homeostatic model assessment (HOMA-IR) and normalized percent of ALA were obtained.

Glucose decreased significantly on the 13 gram intervention compared to the 0.0 gram period [13 g = −2.10 ± 1.66 mg/L (mean ± SEM), 0 g = 9.22 ± 4.44 mg/L]. Insulin decreased significantly on the 13 gram intervention but not the 26 gram and 0.0 gram periods (13 g = −2.12 ± 1.00 mU/L, 26 g = 0.67 ± 0.84 mU/L, 0 g = 1.20 ± 1.16 mU/L). HOMA-IR decreased significantly on the 13 gram period but not on the 26 gram and 0.0 gram periods (13 g = −0.71 ± 0.31, 26 g = 0.27 ± 0.24, 0 g = 0.51 ± 0.35).

The ALA increase for the 0.0 gram period was significantly different from the 13 gram and the 26 gram periods (13 g: 0.20 ± 0.04, 26 g: 0.35 ± 0.07, 0 g: −0.01 ± 0.07). Fructosamine, high-sensitivity C-reactive protein (hCRP), adiponectin and high-sensitivity interleukin-6 showed no significant differences. Flaxseed intake significantly decreased glucose and insulin and improved insulin sensitivity as part of a habitual diet in overweight or obese pre-diabetes individuals. (12)

A meta-analysis published in the journal *Nutrition Reviews* in 2018 aimed to systematically review and analyze randomized controlled trials to determine the effects of flaxseed consumption on glycemic control. The investigators searched PubMed, Medline via Ovid, SCOPUS, Embase and ISI Web of Sciences databases up to November 2016. They selected clinical trials where flaxseed or its products were administered as an intervention.

It was found that there is a significant association between flaxseed supplementation and a reduction in blood glucose, insulin levels and HOMA-IR index, as well as an increase in QUICKI index (see the following). There was no significant impact on HbA1c. In subgroup analysis, a significant reduction in blood glucose, insulin and HOMA-IR and a significant increase in QUICKI were found only in studies using whole flaxseed but not flaxseed oil and lignan extract. Furthermore, a significant reduction was observed in insulin levels and insulin sensitivity indexes only in the subset of trials lasting ≥12 weeks. It was concluded that whole flaxseed, but not flaxseed oil and lignan extract, significantly improves glycemic control. (13)

- *The QUICKI index is a quantitative insulin sensitivity check index, a novel mathematical transformation of fasting blood glucose and insulin levels. It is derived using the inverse of the sum of the logarithms of the fasting insulin and fasting glucose:*

  - *$1 / (\log(\text{fasting insulin } \mu U/mL) + \log(\text{fasting glucose } mg/dL))$*

- *This index correlates well with* glucose clamp *studies, and it is useful for measuring insulin sensitivity, which is the inverse of insulin resistance. It has the advantage that it can be obtained from a fasting blood sample and is the preferred method for certain types of clinical research. (14)*

Another open-labeled clinical trial published in the journal *Clinical Nutrition Research* in 2019 was conducted on patients with type 2 diabetes to investigate the effect of flaxseed-enriched yogurt on glycemic control, lipid profiles and blood pressure. Participants were given 200 grams of 2.5% fat yogurt containing 30 grams of flaxseed, or plain yogurt daily for eight weeks.

After eight weeks of supplementation, HbA1c decreased significantly in the intervention group compared to that in controls. Also, at the end of the study, there were significant differences between the flaxseed-enriched yogurt group and the control groups, in triglycerides and total cholesterol concentrations, systolic blood pressure and diastolic blood pressure.

No significant differences were found between the two groups in low-density lipoprotein, high-density lipoprotein, body weight and waist circumference, and it was therefore concluded that the addition of flaxseed to yogurt can be effective in the management of type 2 diabetes. (15)

Omega-3 fatty acids reduce insulin resistance: A prospective study published in the journal *Annals of Medical Health Sciences Research* in 2013 aimed to determine the effects of antioxidants, e.g., AL, omega-3 fatty acid and vitamin E on parameters of insulin sensitivity (blood glucose and HbA1c) in type 2 diabetes patients with documented insulin resistance. Patients were given ALA, omega 3 fatty acid and vitamin E or just a placebo. Fasting blood glucose and HbA1c were measured at first visit (Visit 1) and after 90 days (Visit 2).

It was found that analysis of baseline (Visit 1) vs. end of treatment period (Visit 2) parameters, showed significant decrease in HbA1c in the three treatment groups. A decrease in fasting blood glucose in the three treatment groups was observed, but it was not statistically significant. The investigators concluded that ALA, omega-3 and vitamin E can be used as "add-on" therapy in patients with type 2 diabetes mellitus to improve insulin sensitivity and lipid metabolism. (23)

A clinical study published in the journal *Scientific Reports* in 2014 aimed to determine whether Omega-3 Index, i.e., red blood cell concentrations of eicosapentaenoic acid (EPA) and docosahexaenoic acid (DHA), affects insulin sensitivity and other metabolic outcomes. The study was conducted on overweight men aged, on average, 46.5 ± 5.1 years.

The participants were assessed twice, 16 weeks apart. Insulin sensitivity was assessed by the Masuda method (55) (see the following) from an oral glucose tolerance test. The participants were separated according to their Omega-3 Index values, e.g., lower tertiles (LOI) and highest tertile (HOI).

Increasing Omega-3 Index was significantly correlated with higher insulin sensitivity, higher disposition index and lower CRP concentrations. Masuda Index insulin sensitivity scores were 43% (significantly) higher in HOI than in LOI men. Similarly, HOI men had a disposition index that was 70% (significantly) higher and fasting insulin concentrations 25% (significantly) lower. HOI men displayed significantly lower nocturnal systolic blood pressure and significantly greater systolic blood pressure dip. Men in the HOI group also had significantly lower concentrations of CRP (41% lower) and significantly lower concentrations of free fatty acids (21% lower).

The investigators concluded that a higher Omega-3 Index is associated with increased insulin sensitivity and a more favorable metabolic profile in middle-aged overweight men. (25)

- *The Masuda Index indicates values that are comparable to the rate of disappearance of plasma glucose measured by* insulin clamp (1mU/kg per min insulin infusion, corrected at the insulin concentration of 100 microU/mL) with glucose tracer.
- *The Disposition Index is the product of insulin sensitivity times the amount of insulin secreted in response to blood glucose levels.*

7.2.1 OMEGA-3 FATTY ACIDS REDUCE TRIGLYCERIDES IN TYPE 2 DIABETES

The aim of another prospective study published in the *Journal of Clinical and Diagnostic Research* in 2017 was to determine the effects of omega-3 fatty acids (derived from fish oil) on lipid profile in type 2 diabetes patients. Patients were assigned to three groups: Group 1 received 500 mg of metformin twice daily and a placebo; Group 2 received 500 mg of metformin twice daily plus 1 gram of omega-3 fatty acids once daily; Group 3 received 500 mg of metformin twice daily and 1 gram of omega-3 fatty acids twice daily.

It was found that Group 2 significantly reduced the triglyceride level from 144.59 ± 14.18 mg/dL to 101 ± 13.31 mg/dL, compared to Group 1, which reduced triglyceride level from 147.67 ± 18.57 mg/dL to 145.8 ± 19.86 mg/dL, respectively. Group 3 receiving 1 gram of omega-3 fatty acids twice daily showed a significant decrease from 144.83 ± 22.17 mg/dL to 86 ± 17.46 mg/dL and was more effective in reducing triglyceride levels than Group 2 receiving only 1 gram of omega-3 fatty acids once daily.

The investigators concluded that omega-3 fatty acids can be given in conjunction with metformin to reduce triglyceride levels in diabetic dyslipidemia without any adverse drug effects or drug interactions. Omega-3 fatty acids were effective in reducing the triglyceride level significantly, as compared to placebo. Two grams of omega-3 fatty acids are, however, more effective than 1 gram in reducing triglyceride levels. (24)

7.2.2 Type 2 Diabetes and Coronary Heart Disease

Type 2 diabetes has been strongly linked to coronary heart disease. Patients with type 2 diabetes are at increased risk of myocardial infarction and stroke. (26) A study published in the *British Journal of Nutrition* in 2019 was performed to determine the effects of vitamin D and omega-3 fatty acids co-supplementation on markers of cardiometabolic risk in diabetic patients with coronary heart disease (CHD). The trial was conducted on vitamin D–deficient diabetic patients with CHD. At baseline, the range of serum 25-hydroxyvitamin D levels in study participants was 6.3–19.9 ng/mL. The participants were assigned to two groups either taking 50,000 IU vitamin D supplements every two weeks plus 1,000 mg omega-3 fatty acids from flaxseed oil or a placebo twice a day for six months.

Vitamin D and omega-3 fatty acids co-supplementation significantly reduced mean and maximum levels of right and left carotid intima-media thickness, compared to the placebo group. The effect of increases in intima-media thickness of the carotid is a sign of cardiovascular disease.

In addition, co-supplementation led to a significant reduction in fasting plasma glucose (β −0·40 mmol/l), insulin (β −1·66 µIU/mL), insulin resistance (β −0·49) and LDL cholesterol (β −0·21 mmol/l), and a significant increase in insulin sensitivity (β + 0·008) and HDL cholesterol (β + 0·09 mmol/L) compared to the placebo group. High-sensitivity CRP (β −1·56 mg/L) was significantly reduced in the supplemented group compared to the placebo group. The investigators concluded that vitamin D and omega-3 fatty acids co-supplementation had beneficial effects on markers of cardiometabolic risk. (27)

7.2.3 Omega-3 Fatty Acid as Adjuvant Treatment of Type 2 Diabetes and Nonalcoholic Fatty Liver Disease (NAFLD)

Nonalcoholic fatty liver disease (NAFLD; steatohepatitis) is rapidly becoming the most common liver disease worldwide. It can progress to liver cirrhosis and, it is thought, even to hepatocarcinoma. The prevalence of NAFLD is 80% to 90% in obese adults, 30% to 50% in patients with diabetes and up to 90% in patients with hyperlipidemia. (29)

The aim of a clinical trial published in the *Chinese Journal of Internal Medicine* (*Zhonghua Nei Ke Za Zhi*) was to determine the relationship between serum omega-3 polyunsaturated fatty acid (omega-3 PUFA) levels and insulin resistance (IR) in patients with type 2 diabetes mellitus and NAFLD. The trial was conducted on patients with type 2 diabetes mellitus with NAFLD (Group 4), patients with type 2 diabetes alone (Group 3), patients with only NAFLD (Group 2) and healthy control participants (Group 1). Serum omega-3 PUFA profile was analyzed with capillary gas chromatography. Insulin resistance was assessed by homeostasis model assessment (HOMA-IR). ALT, AST, gamma-glutamyltransferase (GGT) and serum lipids were measured.

It was found that the levels of HOMA-IR were significantly higher in patients with type 2 diabetes mellitus with NAFLD (Group 4) than those in Group 3 (type 2 diabetes alone), Group 2 (patients with only NAFLD) and Group 1 (control). The levels of ALT, AST, GGT, TC, TG, LDL-C were significantly higher in Group 4 than those in Group 3, Group 2 or Group 1. The level of omega-3 PUFA was significantly lower in Group 4 than those in Groups 3, 2 or 1. Omega-3 PUFA concentration was significantly negatively correlated with HOMA-IR, TC, TG and LDL-C.

The investigators concluded that serum omega-3 PUFA is significantly lowered in patients with type 2 diabetes mellitus and NAFLD. Serum omega-3 PUFA is significantly negatively correlated with insulin resistance. Thus, it can be said that omega-3 PUFA plays a very important role in blunting the development of diabetes mellitus and NAFLD. (30)

7.2.4 Omega-3 Fatty Acid as Adjuvant Treatment of Type 2 Diabetes with Diabetic Nephropathy

The aim of a meta-analysis published in the journal *PlosOne* in 2020 was to evaluate the effects of omega-3 PUFA on proteinuria, estimated glomerular filtration rate (eGFR) and metabolic biomarkers among patients with diabetes. The electronic search included PubMed, Embase and Cochrane Central Register of Controlled Trials from January 1960 to April 2019 to identify randomized control trials, which examined the effects of omega-3 fatty acids on proteinuria, eGFR and metabolic biomarkers among diabetic patients.

It was found that omega-3 fatty acids reduced the amount of proteinuria among type 2 diabetes mellitus to a statistically significant extent. While they also tended to lower proteinuria in type 1 diabetes mellitus patients, the effect was not statistically significant. And only studies where the duration of intervention was 24 weeks or longer demonstrated a significantly lower proteinuria in omega-3 fatty acids treated patients compared to the control group.

There was a higher eGFR in both type 1 and type 2 diabetes groups in omega-3 fatty acids treated patients vs. the control group. However, the effect was not statistically significant.

It was concluded that omega-3 fatty acids could help ameliorate proteinuria in type 2 diabetes with supplementation lasting at least 24 weeks. (31)

A study reported in the *Iran Journal of Kidney Diseases* in 2016 was performed to determine the effects of omega-3 fatty acid supplementation on inflammatory cytokines and advanced glycation end products (AGEs) in patients with diabetic nephropathy (DN). Patients with DN were randomly divided into two groups to receive either 1,000 mg/d of omega-3 fatty acid from flaxseed oil or a placebo for 12 weeks. The primary outcome variables were tumor necrosis factor-α (TNF-α), receptor tumor necrosis factor *alpha* and growth differentiation factor 15. Fasting blood samples were taken at the onset and the end of the study to quantify the related markers.

It was found that, compared to placebo, omega-3 fatty acid supplementation resulted in a significant decrease in serum AGEs (−2.3 ± 2.8 AU versus 0.2 ± 2.5 AU). Despite a significant reduction in serum level of the receptor for AGEs (−0.1 ± 0.3 AU) in the omega-3 fatty acid group, no significant difference was found between the two groups in terms of their effects on the receptor for AGEs. Supplementation with omega-3 fatty acid had no significant effect on the inflammatory cytokines as compared with the placebo. The investigators concluded that omega-3 fatty acid supplementation in patients with diabetic nephropathy had favorable effects on AGEs. (32)

> *AGEs are proteins or lipids that become glycated as a result of exposure to sugars. They are a biomarker implicated in aging and the development, or worsening, of many degenerative diseases, such as diabetes, atherosclerosis and chronic kidney disease.*

7.2.5 Treatment Dosage Matters

There is some disagreement about the possible beneficial effects of omega-3 PUFA supplementation in patients with diabetes and cardiovascular disease. It is likely that conflicting results between different clinical studies and meta-analyses could be due to variable dosage supplementation and supplementation duration, either of which could alter the effects of omega-3 PUFA on cardiometabolic biomarkers.

The authors of a report in 2018, in the journal *Cardiovascular Diabetology*, contend that meta-analyses are commonly limited by the inability to draw inferences regarding dosage, duration and the interaction of dosage and duration of omega-3 PUFA intake. Even so, almost all end points in the so-called negative meta-analyses leaned toward a trend for benefit with a near 10% reduction in cardiovascular outcomes and a borderline statistical significance.

However, many trials included in these meta-analyses tested an insufficient daily dose of omega-3 PUFA of less than 1,000 mg. Probably, the consistent cardiovascular effects of omega-3 PUFA supplements could be expected only with daily doses of more than 2,000 mg. (28)

7.2.6 L-Arginine as Adjuvant Treatment of Type 2 Diabetes—Is Type 2 Diabetes Mellitus an NO Deficiency Disease?

While omega-3 and other constituents of flaxseed and flax oil deliver antioxidants that protect the endothelium, L-arginine (which as we recall is abundant in flax seed) delivers NO, which seems to play a key role in promoting insulin release and overcoming insulin resistance. Recent studies have shown that reduced synthesis of NO from L-arginine in endothelial cells is a major factor contributing to the impaired action of insulin in the vasculature of obese and diabetic people. (51)

The decreased NO generation results from (1) a deficiency of (6R)-5,6,7,8-tetrahydrobiopterin (BH4), (33) an essential cofactor for NO synthase (NOS), and (2) increased generation of glucosamine, an inhibitor of the pentose cycle for the production of NADPH, another cofactor for NOS, from glucose and L-glutamine.

> *A superoxide dismutase-mimetic (tempol) reversed the diabetes mellitus–induced reduction of GTPCH and BH4 and endothelial dysfunction in streptozotocin-induced diabetes mellitus in an animal (rat) model. (33)*

According to a report published in the journal *Biofactors* in 2009, endothelial dysfunction can be prevented by (1) enhancement of BH4 synthesis through supplementation of its precursor (sepiapterin) via the salvage pathway, (2) transfer of the gene for GTP cyclohydrolase-I (the first and key regulatory enzyme for *de novo* synthesis of BH4) or (3) dietary supplementation of L-arginine (which stimulates GTP cyclohydrolase-I expression and inhibits hexosamine production). Modulation of the arginine-NO pathway by BH4 and arginine is beneficial for ameliorating vascular insulin resistance in obesity and diabetes. (34)

Chronic L-arginine supplementation has been shown to improve insulin sensitivity and endothelial function in nonobese type 2 diabetic patients. The aim of a study published in the *American Journal of Physiology, Endocrinology and Metabolism* in 2006 was to determine the effects of a long-term oral L-arginine therapy on adipose fat mass (FM) and muscle free-fat mass (FFM) distribution, daily glucose levels, insulin sensitivity, endothelial function, oxidative stress and adipokine release in obese type 2 diabetic patients with insulin resistance who were treated with a combined regimen of hypocaloric diet and exercise training.

Type 2 diabetes patients who participated in a hypocaloric diet plus an exercise training program for 21 days were divided into two groups: the first group was also treated with 8.3 g/day of L-arginine, and the second group was treated with a placebo.

It was found that body weight, waist circumference, daily glucose profiles, fructosamine, insulin and homeostasis model assessment index significantly decreased in both the diet plus exercise group that received placebo and the diet plus exercise group that received L-arginine. In addition, L-arginine supplementation further significantly decreased FM and waist circumference preserving FFM and significantly improved mean daily glucose profiles and fructosamine.

Additional significant outcomes were a decrease in the area under the curve of cGMP, second messenger of NO; superoxide dismutase, index of antioxidant capacity; and increased adiponectin levels, whereas basal endothelin-1 levels and leptin-to-adiponectin ratio decreased significantly in the L-arginine group.

The investigators concluded that long-term oral L-arginine treatment resulted in an additive effect compared with a diet and exercise training program alone on glucose metabolism and insulin sensitivity. Furthermore, it improved endothelial function, oxidative stress and adipokine release in obese type 2 diabetic patients with insulin resistance. (35)

TNF-α is an inflammatory cytokine produced by macrophages/monocytes during acute inflammation and is responsible for a diverse range of signaling events within cells leading to necrosis or apoptosis. The protein is also important for helping the body fight off infections and cancers.

Diabetes and obesity are very commonly associated metabolic disorders that are linked to chronic inflammation. Leptin is one of the important adipokines released from adipocytes, and its level increases with increasing BMI. TNF-α is released not only by immune cells (macrophages/monocytes) but by adipocytes as well in response to chronic inflammation. Type 2 diabetes mellitus is believed to be associated with low-grade chronic inflammation. (36)

The aim of a study published in the *European Review for Medical and Pharmacological Sciences* journal in 2012 was to determine the influence of L-arginine supplementation on TNF-α, insulin resistance and selected anthropometric and biochemical parameters in patients with visceral obesity. The patients with visceral obesity were randomly assigned to either receive 9 grams of L-arginine or a placebo for three months. Healthy lean participants were used as control. Selected anthropometrical measurements and blood biochemical analyses were performed at baseline and after three months. TNF-α and its soluble receptor 2 (sTNFR2) were assessed in both treated groups. Insulin resistance in the participants was evaluated according to the HOMA-IR protocol.

It was found that the concentration of insulin, TNF-α and sTNFR2 and HOMA-IR levels in obese patients significantly exceeded those observed in the control participants. Basal TNF-α and sTNFR2 concentrations were positively correlated with basal BMI, waist circumference, percent of body fat and HOMA-IR. Furthermore, three-month L-arginine supplementation resulted in a significant decrease in HOMA-IR and insulin concentration. Only an insignificant tendency to decrease TNF-α and sTNFR2 was observed.

The investigators confirmed the role of TNF-α in the complex pathogenesis of insulin resistance in patients with visceral obesity. The three-month, 9-gram L-arginine dose supplementation improved insulin sensitivity in patients with visceral obesity. (37)

The aim of a study published in the journal *Diabetes Care* in 2001 was to determine whether long-term administration of L-arginine acting by normalizing the cGMP pathway could ameliorate peripheral and hepatic insulin sensitivity in lean type 2 diabetic patients.

The study was conducted over a period of three months. In the first month, patients remained on their usual diet; then they were randomly assigned to two groups. In group 1, they were treated with diet plus oral placebo three times per day for two months. In group 2, they were treated for one month with diet plus oral placebo three times per day. Then for one month, they were treated with diet plus 3 grams of L-arginine three times per day.

At the end of the first and the second month, patients underwent a euglycemic-hyperinsulinemic *clamp* combined with [6,6–2H2] glucose infusion.

It was found that in control group 1, there were no changes in basal cGMP levels, systolic blood pressure, forearm blood flow, glucose disposal and endogenous glucose production. In group 2, however, L-arginine normalized basal cGMP levels and significantly increased forearm blood flow by 36% and glucose disposal during the *clamp* by 34%, and it significantly decreased systolic blood pressure and endogenous glucose production by 14% and 29%, respectively. However, compared to that in control participants, the L-arginine treatment did not completely overcome the defect in glucose disposal.

The investigators concluded that L-arginine treatment significantly improves but does not completely normalize peripheral and hepatic insulin sensitivity in type 2 diabetic patients. (38)

What makes these two studies particularly interesting is not only that they demonstrated the benefits of L-arginine in correcting glucose metabolism but that they tied it to the action of NO via the cGMP element of the NO/cGMP pathway.

There is considerable evidence that NO affects insulin release and metabolism, but overall the evidence is controversial. On balance, eNOS-derived NO seems to stimulate insulin release (eNOS is a *constitutive* NOS). On the other hand, *inducible*, i.e., iNOS-derived NO, is said to inhibit insulin secretion. (39, 40) According to a report published in the *EXCLI Journal* in 2020, NO increases insulin secretion. Decreased NO bioavailability has been demonstrated in obesity and type 2 diabetes in both animal and human studies and restoration of NO levels has many favorable metabolic effects in type 2 diabetes, suggesting that NO through modulation of insulin secretion and its signaling pathways may be a potential target for the treatment of type 2 diabetes.

However, some studies have shown that inhibition of islet NO synthase (NOS) activity is accompanied by an increase in glucose-stimulated insulin secretion (GSIS). Moreover, GSIS has been shown to be suppressed by different concentrations of NO-donors, indicating a negative role of NO in insulin secretion.

It is proposed in that report that the controversy over the role of NO in insulin secretion may be artifactual, i.e., that it depends on the use of various β-cell lines with different qualitative/quantitative secretory reaction patterns, incubation of islets/β-cells in high or low glucose media, using different NOS inhibitors or different types of extracellular/intracellular NO-donors. Also varying enzymatic activities of the different isoforms of NOS may be of importance. (41)

Finally, a number of clinical studies have also established the effects of L-arginine supplementation by administering it intravenously. The aim of such a clinical study published in the *European Journal of Clinical Investigation* in 1997 was to determine the effect of a low-dose intravenous supplementation of L-arginine on insulin-mediated vasodilatation and insulin sensitivity.

The study was conducted on healthy participants and on patients with obesity and type 2 diabetes mellitus. Insulin-mediated vasodilatation was measured by venous occlusion plethysmography during the insulin suppression test, evaluating insulin sensitivity. Measurements were obtained twice for each healthy participant and each patient with or without a concomitant infusion of 0.52 mg/kg^{-1} min^{-1} of L-arginine.

L-Arginine significantly restored the impaired insulin-mediated vasodilatation observed in obesity and type 2 diabetes. No significant effect on insulin-mediated vasodilatation was observed in healthy participants. Insulin sensitivity was significantly improved in all groups by infusion of L-arginine. L-Arginine had no effect on insulin, insulin-like growth factor I (IGF-I), free fatty acids (FFAs) or C-peptide levels during the insulin suppression test.

The data show that defective insulin-mediated vasodilatation in obesity and type 2 diabetes can be normalized by intravenous L-arginine: L-arginine improves insulin sensitivity in obese and type 2 diabetes patients, as well as in healthy subjects, suggesting a possible mechanism that is different from the restoration of insulin-mediated vasodilatation. (42)

7.3 FLAX, INFLAMMATION AND ENDOTHELIUM DYSFUNCTION IN CKD

Chronic kidney disease (CKD), also called chronic kidney failure, is the loss of kidney filtration function. The advanced form causes dangerous levels of fluid, electrolytes and wastes to build up in the body. In the early stages of CKD, there may be few signs or symptoms, if any. Treatment centers on slowing the progression of kidney damage, usually by controlling the cause. But even controlling the cause might not keep kidney damage from progressing. CKD can progress to end-stage kidney failure, which is fatal without artificial filtering (dialysis) or a kidney transplant.

According to the Centers for Disease Control and Prevention in "Chronic Kidney Disease in the United States, 2021," 15% of US adults, or 37 million people, are estimated to have CKD. As many as nine in ten adults with CKD do not know they have it, and about two in five adults with severe CKD do not know they have it. (52) Since there is no cure for CKD, what contribution can flaxseed, *per se*, or its relevant constituents, omega-3 fatty acid, L-arginine or cyanogenic glycosides, make to favorably altering the course of the disease? Simply put, CKD shares endothelium dysfunction with cardiovascular diseases that likewise profit from restoring endothelial NO formation.

7.3.1 FLAXSEED AS ADJUVANT TREATMENT OF CKD

There are a number of reports of the beneficial effects of flaxseed, *per se*, on kidney dysfunction, but they are largely based on experimental (animal-model) studies. For instance, a study published in the journal *Kidney International* in 2003 sought to determine whether changing the source of protein intake from animal protein, casein, to plant protein in the form of either soy protein concentrate or flaxseed protein in the diet would have a different impact on renal function and nephropathy in male obese SHR/N-cp rats model (which commonly, as a matter of course, tend to develop diabetes).

The subjects were assigned to one of three diets containing either 20% casein, 20% soy protein concentrate or 20% flaxseed meal. Except for the protein source, all three diets were identical and contained similar amounts of protein, fat, carbohydrates, minerals and vitamins. All animals were maintained on these diets for six months. At the end of the study period, blood sampling and 24-hour urine collections were performed for renal functional measurements, and the kidneys were harvested and examined for histologic evaluation.

It was found that all three groups had similar amounts of food intake and body weight gain and exhibited fasting hyperglycemia and hyperinsulinemia. Plasma glucose levels did not differ among the three groups, but plasma insulin concentration

L-Arginine and Omega-3 Fatty Acids for Type 2 Diabetes and CKD

was significantly lower in rats fed flaxseed meal than those fed either casein or soy protein concentrate. Mean plasma creatinine, creatinine clearance and urinary urea excretion also did not differ significantly between the three groups. By contrast, urinary protein excretion was significantly lower in subjects fed flaxseed than in those fed either casein or soy protein concentrate.

Morphologic analysis of renal structural lesions showed that the percentage of abnormal glomeruli with mesangial expansion and the tubulointerstitial score (an index of severity of tubulointerstitial damage) were significantly reduced in rats fed flaxseed meal compared to those fed casein or soy protein concentrate.

The investigators concluded that dietary protein substitution with flaxseed meal reduces proteinuria and glomerular and tubulointerstitial lesions in obese SHR/N-cp rats and that flaxseed meal is more effective than soy protein in reducing proteinuria and renal histologic abnormalities in this model. The reduction in proteinuria and renal injury was independent of the amount of protein intake and glycemic control. But the investigators could not determine which dietary component(s) present in flaxseed meal is (are) responsible for the renal protective effects. (43)

In another experimental study, this one published in the *Journal of Oleo Science* in 2013, the investigators report that flaxseed-derived PUFAs, including the omega-3 and omega-6 essential fatty acids, have been shown to blunt the effects of hypertension. It is, however, unclear whether the flaxseed, which is rich in these essential fatty acids, could improve the liver and kidney dysfunctions observed in the hypertensive condition. The aim of their study was to examine markers of the liver and kidney function, including aspartate aminotransferase (AST), alanine aminotransferase (ALT), blood urea nitrogen (BUN), uric acid (UA), creatinine and renin in hypertensive male Wistar rats fed a flaxseed diet.

Normotensive subjects maintained on a standard diet were made hypertensive with a daily administration of 25 mg/kg of cyclosporin A (CYS) for four weeks. Subsequently, they were either fed a standard diet alone or a flaxseed-supplemented standard diet (FLX; 10% W/W) for eight weeks.

It was found that compared to normotensive rats, standard diet-fed hypertensive rats had significantly elevated blood pressure, altered lipid profiles and increased plasma levels of tissue markers measured immediately following the CYS treatment and thereafter at four- and eight-week intervals. However, subjects fed the flax-supplemented diet had significantly lower blood pressure and improved lipid profiles after four- and eight-week durations.

The investigators reported that the data demonstrated for the first time the favorable effects of flax in improving liver and kidney functions in the hypertensive condition, and concluded that these effects are likely to result from the ALA contents of flaxseed. (44)

7.3.2 OMEGA-3 FATTY ACIDS IN ADJUVANT TREATMENT OF KIDNEY DISEASE

A report titled "Polyunsaturated Fatty Acids and Renal Fibrosis: Pathophysiologic Link and Potential Clinical Iimplications" was published in the *Journal of Nephrology* in 2005. The authors contend that PUFA may play a key role in renal inflammation and fibrosis, crucial stages in CKD: beneficial effects of omega-3 PUFA on the course of experimental and human nephropathies have been reported.

PUFAs can ameliorate chronic, progressive renal injury beyond the simple reduction of serum lipid levels because they also interfere with the formation of inflammatory factors related both to the modulation of the balance of omega-6- and omega-3-derived eicosanoids and to direct action on the cellular production of the major cytokine mediators of inflammation and on endothelium function.

The mechanisms by which PUFAs can improve some stages in renal fibrosis processes, such as mesangial cell activation and proliferation and extracellular matrix protein synthesis; include the downregulation of some proinflammatory cytokine production, as well as regulation of renin and NO systems; and expression of peroxisome proliferator-activated receptor gene, involved in regulating glucose.

An optimal omega-6/omega-3 PUFA ratio or a high Omega Index dietary intake could offer new therapeutic strategies aimed at interrupting the irreversible process of renal fibrosis and ameliorating chronic renal injury. (16)

A study titled "Blood Omega-3 Fatty Acids Are Inversely Associated with Albumin-Creatinine Ratio in Young and Healthy Adults (The Omega-Kid Study)," published in the journal *Frontiers in Cardiovascular Medicine* in 2021, has important implications for kidney health and disease because an elevated albumin-creatinine ratio (ACR) is a risk factor for cardiovascular disease (CVD), all-cause mortality and accelerated glomerular filtration rate (GFR) decline in the general population.

The investigators aimed to determine the relationship between omega-3 PUFAs and the ACR in healthy individuals with preserved GFR.

The analysis is part of the GAPP study (genetic and phenotypic determinants of blood pressure and other cardiovascular risk factors), a population-based cohort of healthy adults aged 25–41 years. Individuals with known CVD, diabetes or a BMI >35 kg/m2 were excluded. eGFR was calculated according to the combined Creatinine/Cystatin C CKD-EPI formula. ACR was obtained from a fasting morning urine sample. The Omega-3 Index (relative amount of EPA and DHA of total fatty acids in percent) was obtained from whole blood aliquots.

> The Omega-3 Index test is a measure of the amount of EPA and DHA in red blood cell membranes. See https://omegaquant.com/omega-3-index-basic/fpr test kit availability. (53)

A significant inverse relationship was found between the Omega-3 Index and the ACR. No association was found between the Omega-3 Index and eGFR. The adjusted difference in eGFR per 1-unit increase in Omega3-Index was significant (−0.21).

The investigators concluded that a higher Omega-3 Index is significantly associated with lower ACR in this young and healthy population with preserved eGFR. Omega-3 fatty acids may exhibit cardio- and nephroprotective effects in healthy individuals through modulation of the ACR. (17)

Omega-3 fatty acids are associated with a lower risk of CVD and with beneficial effects on CV risk factors. (54) The ACR is a risk factor for CVD, all-cause mortality and accelerated GFR declines in the general population.

The aim of a meta-analysis published in the journal *Clinics* (Sao Paulo) in 2017 was to determine the benefits and/or risks of omega-3 fatty acid supplementation in patients with chronic kidney disease. A systematic search of articles in PubMed, Embase, the Cochrane Library and reference lists was undertaken: all eligible studies assessed proteinuria, the serum creatinine clearance rate, the estimated glomerular filtration rate or the occurrence of end-stage renal disease.

Compared to no-dose or low-dose omega-3 fatty acid supplementation, any or high-dose omega-3 fatty acid supplementation, respectively, was significantly associated with a lower risk of proteinuria but had little or no effect on the serum creatinine clearance rate or the estimated GFR. However, this supplementation was associated with a significantly reduced risk of end-stage renal disease. The investigators concluded that omega-3 fatty acid supplementation is associated with a significantly reduced risk of end-stage renal disease and delays the progression of this disease. (18)

Supplementation of omega-3 fatty acid can ameliorate but not reverse CKD, but such supplementation may be able to avoid it altogether:

Relatively few epidemiological studies have examined the anti-inflammatory properties of PUFA protection against kidney damage in adults. A study published in the *British Journal of Nutrition* in 2011 investigated the association between dietary intakes of PUFA, i.e., omega-3, omega-6, ALA, and fish and the prevalence of CKD. The study examined 2,600 Blue Mountains Eye Study participants 50 years old or older.

> *The Blue Mountains Eye Study is a population-based survey of vision and common eye diseases in residents of a defined area west of Sydney, Australia.*

Dietary data were collected using a semi-quantitative Food Frequency (portion size) Questionnaire (FFQ) and PUFA and fish intakes were calculated. Baseline biochemistry including serum creatinine was measured. Moderate CKD was defined as an estimated glomerular filtration rate of < 60 mL/min per 1.73 m2.

Participants in the highest quartile of long-chain omega-3 PUFA intake had a significantly reduced likelihood of having CKD compared with those in the lowest quartile of intake. The highest, compared with the lowest quartile of fish consumption, was associated with a reduced likelihood of CKD.

The authors concluded that an increased dietary intake of long-chain omega-3 PUFA and fish reduces the prevalence of CKD. They hold that a diet rich in omega-3 PUFA and fish could have a role in maintaining healthy kidney function, in addition to their role in preventing other diseases. (19)

Omega-3 PUFA supplementation may reduce cardiovascular mortality in patients on hemodialysis: another meta-analysis published in the journal *Clinical Nutrition* in 2020 aimed to determine the effects of omega-3 PUFA intake on patients with CKD. The investigators searched Medline, Embase and Central through January 12, 2018. Eligible studies were randomized controlled trials evaluating n-3 PUFA intake (supplementation or dietary) compared with placebo, standard care or other treatment, on cardiovascular and all-cause mortality, end-stage kidney disease (ESKD), acute transplant rejection and allograft loss.

It was found that low to very low certainty evidence suggested that omega-3 PUFA supplementation reduced cardiovascular death for participants on hemodialysis, and prevented ESKD in participants with CKD not receiving renal replacement therapy, but made little or no difference in all-cause mortality, acute transplant rejection or allograft loss.

It was concluded that omega-3 PUFA supplementation may reduce cardiovascular mortality in patients on hemodialysis, but it is uncertain whether supplementation prevents mortality or ESKD in patients with CKD. (20)

Because CKD is typically accompanied by inflammation, a study published in the journal *BioMed Research International* in 2017 aimed to determine the effect of six-month supplementation with omega-3 fatty acids on selected markers of inflammation in patients with CKD stages 1–3: six-month supplementation with 2 grams/day of omega-3 was given to CKD patients and to healthy individuals.

At baseline and after follow-up, blood was taken for CRP and monocyte chemotactic protein-1 (MCP-1) concentration analysis and white blood cell (WBC) count. Serum concentration of omega-3 fatty acids—EPA, DHA and ALA—was determined as well as 24-hour urinary collection was performed to measure MCP-1 excretion.

It was found that after six months of omega-3 supplementation, ALA concentration increased significantly in CKD patients and in the healthy control group, while EPA and DHA did not change. At follow-up, a significant decrease in urinary MCP-1 excretion in CKD and in the reference group was found. CRP, serum MCP-1 and WBC did not change significantly. The estimated glomerular filtration rate (eGFR) did not change significantly in the CKD group.

It was concluded that the reduction in urinary MCP-1 excretion may suggest a beneficial effect of omega-3 supplementation on tubular MCP-1 production. (21)

> *MCP-1 is a potent inflammatory cytokine. It is one of the key chemokines that regulate migration and infiltration of monocytes/macrophages. Migration of monocytes from the bloodstream across the vascular endothelium is required for routine immunological surveillance of tissues, as well as in response to inflammation. (22)*

7.3.3 L-Arginine in Treatment of CKD

As noted earlier, there is considerable attention given to the benefits of omega-3 fatty acids in adjuvant treatment of CKD. The benefits are mostly attributed to promoting endothelium viability. Yet most, albeit not all of the research on L-arginine is conducted on animal models—rats. Investigators are well aware that both diabetes and chronic kidney disease are related insofar as both share endothelium dysfunction. In a sense, then, both are "nitric oxide deficiency diseases" and a number of investigators seem well aware of that.

In a report titled "Arginine, Arginine Analogs and Nitric Oxide Production in Chronic Kidney Disease" published in the journal *Nature Clinical Practice Nephrology* in 2006, the authors make a number of cogent points. They contend that renal disease causes reduced NO production and that this contributes to cardiovascular disease and worsening of kidney damage.

They hold that deficiency of L-arginine and increased levels of circulating endogenous inhibitors of NO synthase (particularly ADMA) cause NO deficiency. The decreased L-arginine availability in CKD is due to perturbed renal biosynthesis of this amino acid. In addition, elevated plasma and tissue levels of ADMA in CKD are due to both reduced renal excretion and reduced catabolism by dimethylarginine dimethylaminohydrolase (DDAH). The latter might be associated with loss-of-function polymorphisms of a DDAH gene, functional inhibition of the enzyme by oxidative stress in CKD and end-stage renal disease or both.

They also aver that there is support for novel therapies, including supplementation of dietary L-arginine or its precursor L-citrulline, the inhibition of non-NO-producing pathways of L-arginine utilization or both. Increased ADMA is now seen as a major independent risk factor in end-stage renal disease (and probably also in CKD), so lowering ADMA concentration might be a major therapeutic goal. (45)

We have raised the issue of excess ADMA formation in a previous section in connection with the "arginine paradox" and also in connection with its excess formation in oxidative stress.

Here is the *Abstract* of a report titled "L-Arginine as a Therapeutic Tool in Kidney Disease" published in the journal *Seminars in Nephrology* in 2004:

Infusion of L-arginine in experimental animals increases renal plasma flow (RPF) and glomerular filtration rate (GFR). It is likely that a component of these hemodynamic changes are mediated by nitric oxide (NO) as suggested by studies with specific antagonists of L-arginine metabolism. L-Arginine administration ameliorates the infiltration of the renal parenchyma by macrophages in rats with obstructive nephropathy or rats with puromycin-induced nephrotic syndrome. L-Arginine administration also blunts the increase in interstitial volume, collagen IV, and alpha-smooth muscle actin. Rats with a remnant kidney given 1% L-arginine in the drinking water had a greater GFR and RPF. L-Arginine administration also decreased proteinuria. Diabetic rats given L-arginine had significantly lower excretion of protein and cyclic guanosine monophosphate than diabetic rats not receiving L-arginine. Despite persistent hyperglycemia, the administration of L-arginine prevented the development of hyperfiltration and ameliorated proteinuria in diabetic rats. In the setting of ischemic acute renal failure, the administration of L-arginine had a beneficial effect on GFR and RPF, decreased O2- production, diminished up-regulation of soluble guanylate cyclase, and prevented up-regulation of inducible NO synthase (iNOS). The pharmacokinetics of L-arginine indicate that side effects are rare and mostly mild and dose dependent. (46) Seminars in Nephrology, with permission.

And, here is yet another example of the recognition of the role of endothelial dysfunction in CKD. It is the *Abstract* of a report titled "Endothelial Dysfunction in Chronic Kidney Disease, from Biology to Clinical Outcomes: A 2020 Update" published in the *Journal of Clinical Medicine* in 2020.

The vascular endothelium is a dynamic, functionally complex organ, modulating multiple biological processes, including vascular tone and permeability, inflammatory responses, thrombosis, and angiogenesis. Endothelial dysfunction is a threat to the integrity of the vascular system, and it is pivotal in the pathogenesis of atherosclerosis and cardiovascular disease. Reduced nitric oxide (NO) bioavailability is a hallmark of chronic kidney disease (CKD), with this disturbance being almost universal in patients who reach the most advanced phase of CKD, end-stage kidney disease (ESKD). Low NO bioavailability in CKD depends on several mechanisms affecting the expression and the activity of endothelial NO synthase (eNOS). Accumulation of endogenous inhibitors of eNOS, inflammation and oxidative stress, advanced glycosylation products (AGEs), bone mineral balance disorders encompassing hyperphosphatemia, high levels of the phosphaturic hormone fibroblast growth factor 23 (FGF23), and low levels of the active form of vitamin D (1,25 vitamin D) and the anti-ageing vasculoprotective factor Klotho all impinge upon NO bioavailability and are critical to endothelial dysfunction in CKD. Wide-ranging multivariate interventions are needed to counter endothelial dysfunction in CKD, an alteration triggering arterial disease and cardiovascular complications in this high-risk population. (47) With permission.

It is clear that we are well aware of the NO-connection in CKD and yet arginine supplementation with a proven track record of enhancing endothelium function is not given the prominence it well deserves.

There are however specific applications of beneficial L-arginine supplementation. For instance: Hypertension may develop in kidney transplant (KT) patients because of reduced NO bioavailability resulting in abnormal NO-mediated vasodilation. Therefore, raising NO bioavailability with L-arginine might restore the NO-mediated vasodilation and lower blood pressure.

The beneficial effects of L-arginine on systemic blood flow have been reported in patients with heart failure and are summarized in another section of this book. But so far, no beneficial effects of L-arginine on systemic blood flow have been reported in connection with those who also suffer from kidney failure. Thus, even if the clinician declines to recommend that these patients take supplemental arginine, they might consider recommending to them that they add flaxseeds to their diet—for the arginine, as well as for the PUFAs and the cyanogenic glycosides.

7.3.4 CKD, Hypertension and Chronic Heart Failure

A study published in the *Journal of Hypertension* in 2000 aimed to determine the effects of oral administration of L-arginine on renal blood flow, sodium and water handling, and various hormonal factors in patients with chronic heart failure. Patients with chronic congestive heart failure (New York Heart Association) Functional Classification II–III, 56 ± 12 years of age) were assigned to receive 15 g/day of oral L-arginine and placebo, or placebo and arginine sequentially for five days each.

Twenty-four-hour creatinine clearance (Ccr), and 24-hour urinary cyclic guanosine 5-monophosphate (cGMP) excretion were determined. Saline loading was performed on day five of each treatment. Renal blood flow, GFR and urinary sodium excretion rate (UNa) were assessed before and after saline loading.

It was found that 24-hour cGMP was significantly higher and plasma endothelin level was significantly lower with L-arginine treatment compared to placebo treatment. In addition, the relative increase of UNa and GFR after saline loading was significantly higher in L-arginine than in placebo treatment.

The investigators concluded that oral administration of L-arginine has beneficial effects on glomerular filtration rate, natriuresis and plasma endothelin level in patients with chronic congestive heart failure. (48)

A prospective pilot study published in JPEN *Journal of Parenteral and Enteral Nutrition* in 2001 reported that normotensive volunteers and KT patients received 9 grams per day of oral L-arginine supplements for nine days; then 18.0 grams per day for nine more days. A group of hemodialysis (HD) and a group of peritoneal dialysis patients received the same dose for 14 days. Some KT patients also received 30 mL/d of canola oil (CanO) in addition to L-arginine. Systolic (SBP) and diastolic (DBP) blood pressure, creatinine clearance (CCr) and serum creatinine (Cr) were measured at baseline, at day nine and at day 18.

In a subsequent study, a group of hypertensive KT patients with stable but abnormal renal function were assigned to a study to start L-arginine-only, or L-arginine + CanO supplements for two 2-month periods with an intervening month of no supplementation. SBP, DBP, CCr and Cr were measured monthly for seven months.

It was found in this pilot study that L-arginine significantly lowered the SBP in HD patients from 171.5 ± 7.5 mm Hg (baseline) to 142.8 ± 8.3 mm Hg. In the crossover study, SBP was significantly reduced from baseline (155.9 ± 5.0 mm Hg), after the first two months (143.2 ± 3.2 mm Hg), and subsequent two months (143.3 ± 2.5 mm Hg) of supplementation. DBP was also reduced after supplementation in both studies. CanO had no effect on blood pressure. Renal function did not change.

The investigators concluded that oral L-arginine supplements and preparations (L-arginine $\pm$ CanO) were well tolerated for up to 60 consecutive days and had favorable effects on systolic and diastolic blood pressure in hypertensive kidney transplant and hemodialysis patients. (49)

Caveat: A study published in the *Journal of the American Society of Nephrology* in 2001 aimed to determine the therapeutic benefits of L-arginine supplementation in allogeneic renal transplantation in Brown Norway rat kidneys transplanted into Lewis rat recipients, with one native kidney remaining. Recipients received 2.5 mg/kg per d low-dose cyclosporin (subcutaneously) to obtain moderate vascular and interstitial rejection, with or without 1% L-arginine in drinking water for seven days post-transplantation.

Transplantation significantly increased renal vasoconstriction thereby reducing GFR. It was found that treatment with L-arginine restored renal graft function to levels found in normal donors. L-Arginine significantly reduced vascular occlusion because of lesser inflammation, endothelial disruption, and thrombosis. L-Arginine also decreased tubulitis, interstitial injury and macrophage infiltration. These protective effects suggest that L-arginine might be useful as additive therapy to conventional immune suppression.

However, there is a downside: the investigators also reported their observation that in a proinflammatory environment, L-arginine can worsen renal injury. (50)

7.4 SUMMARY

Flaxseed yields omega-3, L-arginine and cyanogenic glycosides. The administration of flaxseed *per se*, as well as omega-3 and L-arginine individually as adjuvant treatments have shown benefits in reducing chronic systemic inflammation, promoting insulin secretion in type 2 diabetes and enhancing glomerular filtration in chronic kidney disease. It is the consensus that the beneficial effects of these constituents is the restoration of endothelial function and of NO bioavailability.

There are no published reports of cyanogenic glycosides *per se* in treatment of type 2 diabetes or CKD.

7.5 REFERENCES

1. DeFronzo RA, Ferrannini E, Groop L, Henry RR, Herman WH, Holst JJ, Hu FB, Kahn CR, Raz I, Shulman GI, Simonson DC, Testa MA, and R Weiss. 2015. Type 2 diabetes mellitus. *Nature Reviews Disease Primers*, Jul 23; 1(15019). DOI:10.1038/nrdp.2015.19.
2. Kurtul N, Bakan E, Aksoy H, and O Baykal. 2005. Leukocyte lipid peroxidation, superoxide dismutase and catalase activities of type 2 diabetic patients with retinopathy. *Acta Medica*, 48(1): 35–38. DOI:10.14712/18059694.2018.26.
3. Esterbauer H, Schaur RJ, and H Zollner. 1991. Chemistry and biochemistry of 4-hydroxynonenal, malonaldehyde and related aldehydes. *Free Radical Biology and Medicine*, 11(1): 81–128. DOI:10.1016/0891-5849(91)90192-6.
4. Montonen J, Knekt P, Järvinen R, and A Reunanen. 2004. Dietary antioxidant intake and risk of type 2 diabetes. *Diabetes Care*, Feb; 27(2): 362–366. DOI:10.2337/diacare.27.2.362.
5. No author(s). No date. *Seven Countries Study*. www.sevencountriesstudy.com/glossary2/cross-check-dietary-history/#:~:text=Cross%2Dcheck%20dietary%20history%3A%20A,pattern%20during%20weekdays%20or%20weeks; accessed 11/21/21.
6. Feskens EJM, Virtanen SM, Räsänen L, Tuomilehto J, Stengård J, Pekkanen J, Nissinen A, and D Kromhout. 1995. Dietary factors determining diabetes and impaired glucose tolerance: A 20-year follow-up of the Finnish and Dutch cohorts of the Seven Countries Study. *Diabetes Care*, Aug; 18(8): 1104–1112. DOI:10.2337/diacare.18.8.1104.
7. Tan KCB, Chow W-S, Ai VHG, and KSL Lam. 2002. Effects of angiotensin II receptor antagonist on endothelial vasomotor function and urinary albumin excretion in type 2 diabetic patients with microalbuminuria. *Diabetes/Metabolic Research and Reviews*, Jan–Feb; 18(1): 71–76. DOI:10.1002/dmrr.255.
8. Meigs JB, Hu FB, Rifai N, and JoAE Manson. 2004. Biomarkers of endothelial dysfunction and risk of type 2 diabetes mellitus. *Journal of the American Medical Association (JAMA)*, Apr 28; 291(16): 1978–1986. DOI:10.1001/jama.291.16.1978.
9. Fried R, and RM Carlton. 2018. Type 2 diabetes. In: *Cardiovascular and related complications and evidence-based complementary treatments*. Boca Raton: CRC Press/Taylor & Francis.
10. Mechchate H, Es-safi I, Conte R, Hano C, Amaghnouje A, Jawhari FZ, Radouane N, Bencheikh N, Grafov A, and D Boustal. 2021. In vivo and in vitro antidiabetic and anti-inflammatory properties of flax (*Linum usitatissimum* L.) seed polyphenols. *Nutrients*, Aug; 13(8): 2759. DOI:10.3390/nu13082759.
11. Mani UV, Mani I, Biswas M, and SN Kumar. 2011. An open-label study on the effect of flax seed powder (*Linum usitatissimum*) supplementation in the management of diabetes mellitus. *Journal of Dietary Supplements*, Sep; 8(3): 257–265. DOI:10.3109/19390211.2011.593615.
12. Hutchins AM, Brown BD, Cunnane SC, Domitrovich SG, Adams ER, and CE Bobowiec. 2013. Daily flaxseed consumption improves glycemic control in obese men and women with pre-diabetes: A randomized study. *Nutrition Research*, May; 33(5): 367–375. DOI:10.1016/j.nutres.2013.02.012.
13. Mohammadi-Sartang M, Sohrabi Z, Barati-Boldaji R, Raeisi-Dehkordi H, and Z Mazloom. 2018. Flaxseed supplementation on glucose control and insulin sensitivity:

A systematic review and meta-analysis of 25 randomized, placebo-controlled trials. *Nutrition Reviews*, Feb 1; 76(2): 125–139. DOI:10.1093/nutrit/nux052.
14. Katz A, Nambi SS, Mather K, Baron AD, Follmann DA, Sullivan G, and MJ Quon. 2000. Quantitative insulin sensitivity check index: A simple, accurate method for assessing insulin sensitivity in humans. *Journal of Clinical Endocrinology and Metabolism*, Jul; 85(7): 2402–2410. DOI:10.1210/jcem.85.7.6661.
15. Hasaniani N, Rahimlou M, Ahmadi AR, Khalifani AM, and M Alizadeh. 2019. The effect of flaxseed enriched yogurt on the glycemic status and cardiovascular risk factors in patients with type 2 diabetes mellitus: Randomized, open-labeled, controlled study. *Clinical Nutrition Research*, Oct; 8(4): 284–295. DOI:10.7762/cnr.2019.8.4.284.
16. Baggio B, Musacchio E, and G Priante. 2005. Polyunsaturated fatty acids and renal fibrosis: Pathophysiologic link and potential clinical implications. *Journal of Nephrology*, Jul–Aug; 18(4): 362–327. PMID: 16245238.
17. Filipovic MG, Reiner MF, Rittirsch S, Irincheeva I, Aeschbacher S, Grossmann K, Risch M, Risch L, Limacher A, Conen D, and JH Beer. 2021. Blood omega-3 fatty acids are inversely associated with albumin-creatinine ratio in young and healthy adults (The Omega-Kid Study). *Frontiers in Cardiovascular Medicine*, Apr 27; 8: 622619. DOI:10.3389/fcvm.2021.622619.
18. Hu J, Liu Z, and H Zhang. 2017. Omega-3 fatty acid supplementation as an adjunctive therapy in the treatment of chronic kidney disease: A meta-analysis. *Clinics (Sao Paulo)*, Jan; 72(1): 58–64. DOI:10.6061/clinics/2017(01)10.
19. Gopinath B, Harris DC, Flood VM, Burlutsky G, and P Mitchell. 2011. Consumption of long-chain n-3 PUFA, α-linolenic acid and fish is associated with the prevalence of chronic kidney disease. *British Journal of Nutrition*, May; 105(9): 1361–1368. DOI:10.1017/S0007114510005040.
20. Saglimbene VM, Wong G, van Zwieten A, Palmer SC, Ruospo M, Natale P, Campbell K, Teixeira-Pinto A, Craig JC, and GFM Strippoli. 2020. Effects of omega-3 polyunsaturated fatty acid intake in patients with chronic kidney disease: Systematic review and meta-analysis of randomized controlled trials. *Clinical Nutrition*, Feb; 39(2): 358–368. DOI:10.1016/j.clnu.2019.02.041.
21. Pluta A, Stróżecki P, Kęsy J, Lis K, Sulikowska B, Odrowąż-Sypniewska G, and J Manitius. 2017. Beneficial effects of 6-month supplementation with omega-3 acids on selected inflammatory markers in patients with chronic kidney disease Stages 1–3. *BioMed Research International*, 2017: 1680985. DOI:10.1155/2017/1680985.
22. Deshmane SL, Kremlev S, Amini S, and BE Sawaya. 2010. Monocyte chemoattractant protein-1 (MCP-1): An overview. *Journal of Interferon and Cytokine Research*, 29(6). DOI:10.1089/jir.2008.0027.
23. Udupa A, Nahar P, Shah S, Kshirsagar M, and B Ghongane. 2013. A comparative study of effects of omega-3 fatty acids, alpha lipoic acid and vitamin E in type 2 diabetes mellitus. *Annals of Medical Health Sciences Research*, Jul; 3(3): 442–446. DOI:10.4103/2141-9248.117954.
24. Chauhan S, Hanish Kodali H, Noor J, Ramteke K, and V Gawai. 2017. Role of omega-3 fatty acids on lipid profile in diabetic dyslipidaemia: Single blind, randomised clinical trial. *Journal of Clinical and Diagnostic Research*, Mar; 11(3): OC13–OC16. DOI:10.7860/JCDR/2017/20628.9449.
25. Albert BB, Derraik JGB, Brennan CM, Biggs JB, Smith GC, Garg ML, Cameron-Smith D, Hofman PL, and WS Cutfield. 2014. Higher omega-3 index is associated with increased insulin sensitivity and more favourable metabolic profile in middle-aged overweight men. *Scientific Reports*, Oct 21; 4: 6697. DOI:10.1038/srep06697.
26. Shah AD, Langenberg C, Rapsomaniki E, Spiros Denaxas S, Pujades-Rodriguez M, Gale CP, Deanfield J, Smeeth L, Timmis A, and H Hemingway. 2015. Type 2 diabetes

and incidence of cardiovascular diseases: A cohort study in 1·9 million people. *Lancet, Diabetes and Endocrinology*, Feb; 3(2): 105–113. DOI:10.1016/S2213-8587(14)70219-0.
27. Talari HR, Najafi V, Raygan F, Mirhosseini N, Ostadmohammadi V, Amirani E, Taghizadeh M, Hajijafari M, Shafabakhsh R, and Z Asemi. 2019. Long-term vitamin D and high-dose n-3 fatty acids' supplementation improve markers of cardiometabolic risk in type 2 diabetic patients with CHD. *British Journal of Nutrition*, Aug 28; 122(4): 423–430. DOI:10.1017/S0007114519001132.
28. Tenenbaum A, and EZ Fisman. 2018. Omega-3 polyunsaturated fatty acids supplementation in patients with diabetes and cardiovascular disease risk: Does dose really matter? *Cardiovascular Diabetology*, 17: 119. DOI:10.1186/s12933-018-0766-0.
29. Bellentani S, Scaglioni F, Marino M, and G Bedogni. 2010. Epidemiology of non-alcoholic fatty liver disease. *Digestive Diseases* (Basel Switzerland), 28(1): 155–161. DOI:10.1159/000282080.
30. Zhu Q-Q, Lou D-J, Si X-W, Guan L-L, You Q-Y, Yu Z-M, Zhang A-Z, and D Li. 2010. [Serum omega-3 polyunsaturated fatty acid and insulin resistance in type 2 diabetes mellitus and non-alcoholic fatty liver disease. Article in Chinese], *Zhonghua Nei Ke Za Zhi* (*Chinese Journal of Internal Medicine*), Apr; 49(4): 305–308. PMID: 20627036.
31. Chewcharat A, Chewcharat P, Rutirapong A, and S Papatheodorou. 2020. The effects of omega-3 fatty acids on diabetic nephropathy: A meta-analysis of randomized controlled trials. *PLoS ONE*, 15(2): e0228315. DOI: https://doi.org/ 10.1371/journal.pone.0228315.
32. Mirhashemi SM, Rahimi F, Soleimani A, and Z Asemi. 2016. Effects of omega-3 fatty acid supplementation on inflammatory cytokines and advanced glycation end products in patients with diabetic nephropathy: A randomized controlled trial. *Iran Journal of Kidney Diseases*, Jul; 10(4): 197–204. PMID: 27514766.
33. Xu J, Wu Y, Song P, Zhang M, Wang S, and M-H Zou. 2007. Proteasome-dependent degradation of guanosine 5′-triphosphate cyclohydrolase I causes tetrahydrobiopterin deficiency in diabetes mellitus. *Circulation*, 116(8): 944–953. https://doi.org/10.1161/circulationaha.106.684795.
34. Wu G, and CJ Meininger. 2009. Nitric oxide and vascular insulin resistance. *Biofactors*, Jan–Feb; 35(1): 21–27. DOI:10.1002/biof.3.
35. Lucotti P, Setola E, Monti LD, Galluccio E, Costa S, Sandoli EP, Fermo I, Rabaiotti G, Gatti R, and P-M Piatti. 2006. Beneficial effects of a long-term oral l-arginine treatment added to a hypocaloric diet and exercise training program in obese, insulin-resistant type 2 diabetic patients. *Journal of Physiology, Endocrinology and Metabolism*, Nov 1; 291(5): E906—E912. 2006. DOI: https://doi.org/10.1152/ ajpendo.00002.2006.
36. Alzamil H. 2020. Elevated serum TNF-α is related to obesity in type 2 diabetes mellitus and is associated with glycemic control and insulin resistance. *Journal of Obesity*, 2020(5076858): DOI:10.1155/2020/5076858.
37. Bogdanski P, Suliburska J, Grabanska K, Musialik K, Cieslewicz A, Skoluda A, and A Jablecki. 2012. Effect of 3-month L-arginine supplementation on insulin resistance and tumor necrosis factor activity in patients with visceral obesity. *European Review for Medical and Pharmacological Sciences*, Jun; 16(6): 816–823. PMID: 22913215.
38. Piatti PM, Monti LD, Valsecchi G, Magni F, Setola E, Marchesi F, Galli-Kienle M, Guido Pozza G, and KGMM Alberti. 2001. Long-term oral L-arginine administration improves peripheral and hepatic insulin sensitivity in type 2 diabetic patients. *Diabetes Care*, May; 24(5): 875–880. DOI:10.2337/diacare.24.5.875.
39. Nystrom T, Ortsater H, Huang Z, Zhang F, Larsen FJ, Weitzberg E, Lundberg JO, and A Sjöholm. 2012. Norganic nitrite stimulates pancreatic islet blood flow and insulin secretion. *Free Radical Biology and Medicine*, Sep 1; 53: 1017–1023. DOI:10.1016/j.freeradbiomed.2012.06.031.

40. Sansbury BE, and BG Hill. 2014. Regulation of obesity and insulin resistance by nitric oxide. *Free Radical Biology and Medicine*, Aug; 73: 383–399. DOI:10.1016/j.freeradbiomed.2014.05.016.
41. Gheibi S, and A Ghasemi. 2020. Insulin secretion: The nitric oxide controversy. *EXCLI Journal*, 19: 1227–1245. DOI:10.17179/excli2020-2711.
42. Wascher TC, Graier WF, Dittrich P, Hussain MA, Bahadori B, Wallner SJ, and H Toplak. 1997. Effects of low-dose l-arginine on insulin-mediated vasodilatation and insulin sensitivity. *European Journal of Clinical Investigation*, 27(Corpus ID: 23867877). DOI:10.1046/j.1365-2362.1997.1730718.x.
43. Velasquez MT, Bhathena SJ, Ranich T, Schwartz AM, Kardon DE, Ali AA, Haudenschild CC, and CT Hansen. 2003. Dietary flaxseed meal reduces proteinuria and ameliorates nephropathy in an animal model of type II diabetes mellitus. *Kidney International*, Dec; 64(6): 2100–2107. DOI:10.1046/j.1523-1755.2003.00329.x.
44. Al-Bishri WM. 2013. Favorable effects of flaxseed supplemented diet on liver and kidney functions in hypertensive Wistar rats. *Journal of Oleo Science*, 62(9): 709–715. DOI:10.5650/jos.62.709.
45. Baylis C. 2006. Arginine, arginine analogs and nitric oxide production in chronic kidney disease. *Nature Clinical Practice Nephrology*, Apr; 2(4): 209–220. DOI:10.1038/ncpneph0143.
46. Klahr S, and J Morrissey. 2004. L-Arginine as a therapeutic tool in kidney disease. *Seminars in Nephrology*, Jul; 24(4): 389–394. DOI:10.1016/j.semnephrol.2004.04.010.
47. Roumeliotis S. Mallamaci F, and C Zoccali. 2020. Endothelial dysfunction in chronic kidney disease, from biology to clinical outcomes: A 2020 update. *Journal of Clinical Medicine*, Aug; 9(8): 2359. DOI:10.3390/jcm9082359.
48. Watanabe G, Tomiyama H, and N Doba. 2000. Effects of oral administration of L-arginine on renal function in patients with heart failure. *Journal of Hypertension*, Feb; 18(2): 229–234. DOI:10.1097/00004872-200018020-00015.
49. Kelly BS, Alexande JW, Dreyer D, Greenberg NA, Erickson A, Whiting JF, Ogle CK, Babcock GF, and MR First. 2001. Oral arginine improves blood pressure in renal transplant and hemodialysis patients. *JPEN Journal of Parenteral and Enteral Nutrition*, Jul–Aug; 25(4): 194–202. DOI:10.1177/0148607101025004194.
50. Vos IHC, Rabelink TJ, Dorland B, Loos R, van Middelaar B, Grone H-J, and JA Joles. 2001. L-Arginine supplementation improves function and reduces inflammation in renal allografts. *Journal of the American Society of Nephrology*, Feb; 12(2): 361–367. DOI:10.1681/ASN.V122361.
51. Kolluru GK, Bir SC, and CG Kevil. 2012. Endothelial dysfunction and diabetes: Effects on angiogenesis, vascular remodeling, and wound healing. *International Journal of Vascular Medicine*, 2012: 918267. DOI:10.1155/2012/918267.
52. www.cdc.gov/kidneydisease/publications-resources/ckd-national-facts.html; accessed 11/23/21.
53. Harris WS, von Schacky C, and Y Park. 2013. Standardizing methods for assessing omega-3 biostatus. In: McNamara RK, ed. *The omega-3 deficiency syndrome*. Hauppauge, NY: Nova Publishers, pp. 385–398.
54. Harris WS, and C Von Schacky. The omega-3 index: A new risk factor for death from coronary heart disease? *Preventive Medicine*, Jul; 39(1): 212–220. DOI:10.1016/j.ypmed.2004.02.030.
55. Masuda H, and A Matsuoka. 1997. Advances in clinical laboratory tests for diabetes mellitus. *Rinsho Byori (Japanese Journal of Clinical Pathology)*, Sep; 45(9): 844–849. PMID: 9311257.

8 NO from Flaxseed Enhances Sexual Function

8.1 PROLOGUE

Flaxseed has a number of important properties that directly lead to maintaining sexual "health," even enhancing sexual function throughout maturity. First, flaxseed delivers L-arginine, a nitric oxide (NO)-donor. Why that is important will be explained in the following sections of this chapter. Second, it delivers cyanogenic glycosides (CNglcs), likewise NO-donors. Third, it contains high levels of the antioxidant omega-3 fatty acid alpha-linolenic acid (ALA) that has been shown to protect the endothelium, even enhancing endothelial nitric oxide (eNO) formation where and when it is needed in the body.

For instance, flaxseeds (and flax oil) contain a group of nutrients called lignans, which have powerful antioxidant and estrogenic properties. (30) The lignans are a large group of polyphenols found in plants, particularly seeds, whole grains and vegetables. Lignans are precursors to phytoestrogens. Free radicals and the commonly resulting reactive oxygen species (ROS) are the very bane of eNO formation. The surest way to jeopardize eNO formation is an antioxidant-poor diet.

Flaxseed does not promote an increase in free testosterone levels; it reduces androgen levels in both men and women. This reduction may possibly retard or slow down the process of hair loss called pattern baldness (alopecia) because it prevents testosterone from converting to the more potent dihydrotestosterone, a powerful androgen implicated in that process. (29)

8.2 THE OYSTER AND THE BLUE PILL: SEXUAL *DESIRE* VS. SEXUAL *PERFORMANCE*

Contrary to everything that has been said about different kinds of aphrodisiacs that one can take to increase sexual desire (libido), science tells us that, with few exceptions, the only real biological fuel for sexual desire is the steroid hormone *testosterone*. The countless alleged aphrodisiacs, including foods—oysters come to mind—beverages, salves and amulets that we hear and read about that are said to increase desire usually fail because they don't raise testosterone levels. Even the expectation—the *placebo* effect, as it were—that these will improve performance by increasing desire usually falls short of fulfillment.

We have been consistently led to confuse desire with performance, reasoning that if performance is inadequate, it must be due to lacking desire. It's the old adage, "You could if you wanted to." And so, we have witnessed a search for aphrodisiacs spanning recorded history. Sometimes that search comes with a twist.

8.2.1 What We Learn from *The Perfumed Garden of the Shaykh Nefzawi*

Abou el Heidja has deflowered in one night
Once eighty virgins, and he did not eat nor drink between
Because he'd surfeited himself first with chick'peas
And had drunk camel's milk with honey mixed."

(ca. 15th Century) R. Burton Translation

In the translation by Sir Richard Burton of the 15th-century tome on sexuality, it is reported that Abou el Heidja had deflowered in one night once 80 virgins because he'd surfeited himself first with chick'peas [ibid.]. It so happens that while chickpeas are not notably aphrodisiacs, they do proffer a considerable amount of L-arginine, a key NO-donor necessary for satisfactory "performance":

In a typical serving size of 1 cup of chickpeas (or 200 grams), there are 3.64 grams of L-arginine. That's a lot and, by the way, enough to avoid if one has an active *herpes* infection. For that reason, the previous book of the first author, *Great Food/Great Sex. The Three Food Factors for Sexual Fitness* (Time/Warner Books, 2006) cites chickpeas among foods highly recommended to enhance sexual performance.

Parenthetically, and much to the chagrin of those who mistakenly think that fat is fattening, the only "food" that is reliably aphrodisiac, in a sense, is fat, of course. Because testosterone is a steroid hormone derived from cholesterol, changes in fat intake can alter testosterone levels.

In a study published in the *Journal of Steroid Biochemistry and Molecular Biology*, in 2021, low-fat diets were reported to decrease testosterone levels in men. Men with North American and European ancestry experienced a greater decrease in testosterone in response to a low-fat diet. This study first put men on a high-fat diet (40% fat) and then transferred them to a low-fat diet (20% fat), and found their testosterone levels decreased by 10%–15% on average. Vegetarian low-fat diets caused decreases in testosterone levels up to 26%. Men on high-fat diets had testosterone levels that were about 60 points higher, on average, than men on low-fat diets. (31)

Modern science, however, does not support the reasoning that, *ipso facto*, low performance means low desire. In fact, while sexual performance commonly follows desire, it can also be quite independent of desire, although it is true that we commonly engage in sex when we desire to do so. But up to now, most people who experience consistent failure of performance may attribute it, as psychoanalysts falsely claim, to subconscious sabotage of desire. We know better now. Inadequate performance is commonly a medical issue, although it may ultimately cause a psychological problem.

8.3 THE MOST COMMON CAUSE OF ERECTILE DYSFUNCTION

While a great many American men—said to exceed 30 million—suffer varying degrees of erectile dysfunction (ED), their problem is rarely low or absent sexual desire. American men would not resort to, and pay the high cost of prescription meds such as Viagra® and Cialis® for instance, if they had no desire for sex. The millions of such prescriptions filled by consumers tell us clearly that their problem is weak or absent sexual *performance*—absent or unreliable penile erection—not *lack of desire*: they want to do it . . . but somehow, they can't.

In the past, ED in adult men was most often, and erroneously, blamed on weak or absent *desire* (low or absent libido) due to subconscious psychological issues. The emotional basis of ED was steeped in Freudian *psychobabble* about subconscious *oedipal* conflict and similar myths. This explanation had enjoyed great popularity in the United States despite the lack of any shred of evidence to support it.

Men who think the secret to addressing ED is rooted in emotional problems might consider the following: according to the National Institutes of Health (NIH), about 4% of men in their 50s, and nearly 17% of men in their 60s, experience a total inability to achieve an erection. The incidence jumps to 47% for men older than 75 (see National Institutes of Health [NIH] Consensus Conference. NIH Consensus Development Panel on Impotence. *JAMA*, 1993).

Judging from these statistics, one would have to conclude that in a fair number of American men, subconscious emotional conflicts lie in wait, hidden out of sight, until their mid-50s and 60s when they suddenly surge as would an epidemic simultaneously now infecting almost half the population of men, and completing the infection by the time they reach the age of 75. There is neither logic nor any scientific basis for concluding that subconscious psychological conflicts develop and grow in severity as we mature until, in our middle years, they finally worsen and bring us down.

It could, of course, be that sexual desire declines with age because testosterone, the "hormone of desire," declines with advancing age. While that is certainly true, it is not generally the case that serum available testosterone levels decline precipitously in the middle years, as shown in a later section of this chapter.

In fact, age-related change causes an enzyme, 5α-reductase, to convert testosterone to an even more powerful form, dihydrotestosterone (DHT), that boosts desire (libido) and, by the way, causes benign prostate hypertrophy (BPH), as well as *pattern baldness*. We do however know now that there is an age-related decline in NO production that would directly affect performance.

Conventional medical treatment for either BPH or pattern baldness, parenthetically; or both, consists mainly of prescription meds that inhibit the action of the enzyme, 5α-reductase (for instance, Dutasteride®). These are however not without some risk of adverse impact on libido and erectile function: in 2012, the *Journal of Sexual Medicine* reported that Finasteride (Propecia®) has been associated with sexual side effects that may persist despite discontinuation of the medication. In a clinical series, 20% of subjects with male pattern hair loss had persistent sexual dysfunction for more than six years, suggesting the possibility that the dysfunction may be permanent. (1)

While libido in men and in women depends almost entirely on testosterone, it does not fuel performance. The average testosterone level of men between the ages of 59 and 69 is somewhat lower than that in men between 19 and 29. The concentration of plasma testosterone is quite variable (2) with the highest levels and least variability in men between the ages of 32 and 51. But even by the age of 70, while more variable and thus less predictable, testosterone levels are not all that low. (3) Free-form testosterone does decline with age, but it is not dramatically lower until about age 80.

In 2009, Americans spent $807.7 million on erection-promoting prescription meds. Why would they do that if they lacked sexual desire?

8.4 GAS FUELS PERFORMANCE

Testosterone fuels desire but the gas NO fuels performance. As you will see, bottom line, no matter how much testosterone is there to fuel desire, if the body can't come up with an adequate supply of NO where and when needed, performance suffers. So, to understand why a NO-donor like flaxseed can improve—even restore—sexual performance, it helps to know a little about what science calls the "ACh/NO/cGMP pathway."

In the early 1900s, the Austrian pharmacologist Otto Loewi discovered an interesting substance made by nerve cells in the brain and in the body. Some years later, Sir Henry Dale, with whom Loewi later collaborated at the University of London, and with whom he shared the 1936 Nobel Prize in Medicine named it "acetylcholine" (ACh). This was the beginning of modern neuropharmacology based on chemical signals called *neurotransmitters* by which cells in the nervous system and brain communicate.

ACh was found to relax the arterial smooth muscles all throughout the circulatory system, and this seemed a promising road to lower blood pressure to treat hypertension. However, it did so unreliably and unpredictably. No one knew why.

In 1980, Dr. Robert F. Furchgott, professor of pharmacology at Downstate Medical Center in Brooklyn, New York, published his findings in the journal *Nature* that ACh relaxation of arterial smooth muscle depended on the simultaneous presence of a mysterious substance actually made by the *endothelium*, the inner lining of those blood vessels. The endothelium is an accordion-like structure lining the inner surface of the arterial blood vessels. There is an illustration of the endothelium in Chapter 3 (see Figure 3.2 colored scanning electron micrograph [SEM] of a sectioned artery containing red blood cells).

The mysterious substance was initially termed *"endothelium-derived relaxing factor"* (EDRF): ACh relaxed the blood vessels only when EDRF was also present (4). No one had any idea what EDRF actually was.

It did not take long to verify the finding, and in 1993, Dr. Salvador Moncada at Wellcome Research Labs, United Kingdom, first identified EDRF as a gas, NO, and detailed its role in health and disease in the *New England Journal of Medicine* (NEJM) (5). NO is derived in the body principally from the food-borne amino acid L-arginine and from dietary nitrates as well. At first, this news was, of course, met with disbelief—even derision. A gas, indeed! It was not known then that NO had a biological role, much less in blood vessels.

Then, in 1998, Dr. Furchgott and two colleagues were awarded the Nobel Prize in Medicine for the discovery of the biological role of NO in blood vessels and heart function, and in the nervous system and the brain. The immune system was soon added to the list of NO-dependent body systems.

One of the three recipients, Dr. Louis J. Ignaro, detailed how in sexual arousal, ACh led to increased and sustained production of NO made from the amino acid L-arginine by the endothelium lining the spongy chambers of the penis cavernosa(e) (see the following section). This causes them to relax (dilate) allowing increase blood inflow and, thus, erection.

8.4.1 How a Simple "Blunder" Explains Cardiovascular and Heart Disease

When the body forms Ach, it should invariably cause the formation of NO by the endothelium of arterial blood vessels, causing them to relax and increase blood flow. So why didn't it do that reliably in Dr. Furgott's laboratory?

What Dr. Furchgott discovered in strips of arterial blood vessels washed with Ach is that the strips did not relax when, on closer examination, it was found that laboratory preparation had damaged the endothelium. A simple blunder, perhaps, but it was soon learned that damaged endothelium can't form NO. And this turned out to be a very important lesson for medicine with far-reaching implications for cardiovascular health and for the treatment of ED as well.

The observation that damaged endothelium can't produce NO in amounts sufficient to cause blood vessel dilation and maintain adequate blood circulation is the explanation for how we come by cardiovascular disorders such as hypertension, atherosclerosis, heart failure, kidney disease and metabolic syndrome, and now we can add ED.

Each of these conditions is said to result from damage to the endothelium, and each, in turn, causes further damage to the endothelium. But in the population at risk, it is diet and lifestyle factors—especially a low antioxidants diet—that damage the endothelium and not some laboratory blunder.

8.5 THE CULPRIT: OXIDATIVE STRESS

Although we are entirely dependent on oxygen for survival, our body limits how much we absorb because in fact, in excess, we would actually burn up, i.e. oxidize. But that's not the worst of it. In its common form, O_2 sustains life. But if you tamper with its molecular structure, it can become an unstable "free radical" that destabilizes everything it comes into contact with, creating new and toxic compounds that we call *reactive oxygen species* (ROS). Oxidized lipoprotein and hydrogen peroxide are examples of ROS formed in the body by oxygen free radicals formed, actually, by our own metabolism.

There are also always oxygen free radicals in the surrounding air. So, if you leave an apple exposed to air, for instance, it will shrivel and turn brown, resulting in a new species of apple, *rotten*. Likewise, butter left exposed on the kitchen counter metamorphoses from fresh to a new species of butter, *rancid*. Lipids circulating in the bloodstream are typically safe until they combine with oxygen free radicals forming new, reactive species. These are very appetizing to white blood cells (macrophages) that readily gobble them up and infiltrate blood vessel walls to form atherosclerosis.

Oxidative stress is the cost to the body of an imbalance between ROS and the ability of the body to detoxify with antioxidants and to repair the resulting damage. What are the main precursors of oxidative stress? Recapitulating, factors that may increase a person's risk of long-term oxidative stress include

- Obesity
- Diets high in saturated fats, sugar and processed foods
- Exposure to radiation
- Smoking cigarettes or other tobacco products
- Alcohol consumption
- Certain medications
- Pollution
- Exposure to pesticides or industrial chemicals

Oxidative stress impairs endothelium function as surely as if it were mechanically damaged by mishandling—as in Dr. Furchgott's laboratory. And, by the way, high on the list of contributors to oxidative stress is the high salt, high sugar, high saturated fat, low antioxidant Standard American Diet (SAD).

It bears mention that while the damage to the endothelium in Dr. Furchgott's lab was thought due to "careless handling, "careless" is not really accurate because, at that time, no one had any idea that the endothelium had any vital biological control function, so why spare it? It was thought then to be not much more than a sort of inert lining between the bloodstream and the blood vessel walls to keep undesirable stuff in blood out of the vessel walls.

So, let's look at the endothelium and the part it plays in translating sexual arousal into sexual performance via the so-called Ach/NO/cGMP pathway.

8.6 THE ENDOTHELIUM FORMS NITRIC OXIDE (eNO)

Arterial blood vessels have three major structures: the outer wall composed of smooth muscle rings that surround the blood vessels: these can constrict (narrowing them) or relax (dilating them), a middle wall and the inner cell lining, or endothelium. In ordinary circumstances, the degree of constriction, or *tonus*, of arterial blood vessels, and consequently blood pressure, is principally determined by activity level in two control signal systems:

- The endothelium-dependent signal system based on the availability of L-arginine-derived NO, produced by the endothelium, and
- The endothelium-independent system of action-hormones (adrenaline, noradrenalin, etc.) and by diuresis regulating body sodium levels.

There are others, but these dominate.

As previously noted, the endothelium is a thin layer of cells lining the interior surface of blood vessels. It shields the vessel wall from circulating blood in the vessel inner cavity through which blood flows called the *lumen*. Endothelial cells line the entire circulatory system from the heart to the smallest capillary. They reduce the turbulence of blood flowing through the vessel, allowing it to be pumped farther. These cells also function in vasoconstriction and vasodilation, and hence they control blood flow and pressure.

The endothelium has a barrier function: it acts as a selective barrier between the vessel lumen and surrounding tissue, controlling the passage of materials and the passage of white blood cells into and out of the bloodstream.

8.6.1 THE GLYCOCALYX: SUGAR COATING THE ENDOTHELIUM

Most descriptions of blood vessels, including the endothelium, portray the endothelium as lining the inner surface of the blood vessel so that blood coursing through the lumen comes in direct contact with it. That is actually not the case. The surface of the endothelium facing blood flow has a microscopic "sugar coating" called the glycocalyx that insulates it and protects it from damaging substances such as bacteria and viruses in the bloodstream. Damage to the glycocalyx typically results in damage to the endothelium, impairing its ability to form NO where and when needed. This is significant not only to our understanding of cardiovascular and heart disease but also to erectile function, as well as ED.

For instance, excess salt in diet damages the glycocalyx (6), and so does diabetes. (7) It is also thought to contribute to hypertension (8) and to lead to the formation of atherosclerosis. (9) These are all the well-known cardiovascular and heart hazards that are also associated with ED. And it should come as no surprise that the glycocalyx is often found to be damaged as a result of COVID-19 infection. (10)

Damage to the glycocalyx subjects the endothelium to shear stress as blood courses over it under pressure. This stress on the endothelium also contributes to its impairment of NO formation. (11) That the damage to the glycocalyx leaves the endothelium vulnerable to assault may go a long way to explain the "cardiovascular" complications of both COVID-19 infection and those leading to ED.

The ability of the endothelium to deliver NO in sexual arousal is the key to erectile function and thus satisfactory sexual performance because it is NO that is needed in the "pathway" for the blood vessel to relax. The *endothelium* is the gateway to sexual "performance" vitality, and the glycocalyx protects the endothelium and thus protects NO formation where and when needed to assure that vitality.

8.7 SEXUAL PERFORMANCE IS ABOUT *SHUNTING* BLOOD FLOW IN THE BODY

In old-fashioned railroad parlance, "shunting" meant to move a train from the main line to a siding. Sexual performance requires the shunting of blood from the main circulation in the body to the sex organs: the body is the main line, and the sex organs are the siding. There is a good reason for that.

In ordinary circumstances, most people are not consistently in a state of sexual arousal: in men, the penis is flaccid. That means that blood is flowing through it, but not in sufficient volume to cause and maintain erection. In women, blood is likewise flowing through the clitoris and the labia but not in sufficient volume to cause and maintain engorgement. So, to begin with, sexual arousal can result in, at best, a transient physical state because nature intended it to be transient. Nature invested more in supplying blood to the organs of the body that keep us alive and active than to those that involve reproduction.

How does the shunting mechanism work? Let's first look at the parts and then at how they work in sequence in sexual response.

8.7.1 The Penis Is Not a Muscle

How NO affects blood vessels and what this has to do with erection makes sense only if one understands that the penis is basically a bundle of blood vessels. There are, of course, muscles at the base of the penis, those attached to the pelvis by means of which most men can slightly raise an erect penis. But the penis is largely an encased pair of spongy "cavernosa" chambers—side by side—that are, in fact, modified, spongy arterial blood vessels with blood-supplying arteries whose endothelium controls blood inflow.

Figure 8.1 shows a transverse section of the penis: The two large central spongy *corpora cavernosae*, as well as a spongy chamber that encircles the urethra, the *corpora spongeosum*. The blood inflow cavernosal arteries are shown in the chambers. These engorge with blood during sexual stimulation with increased NO signaling the endothelium to relax the vessel.

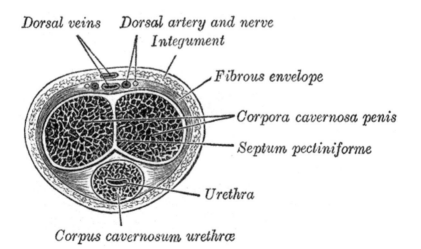

FIGURE 8.1 Cross-section of the penis. (From https://en.wikipedia.org/wiki/Corpus_cavernosum_penis#/media/File:Gray1155.png.)

As the penis erects, the bulging chambers constrict the veins under the relatively inelastic outer *tunica*, thus causing less blood to flow out of the penis through the veins than comes into it through the arteries: this is basically a pressure regulated mechanical valve controlled by a biologically active gas.

8.8 THE (ACh/NO/cGMP) PATHWAY TO PENILE ERECTION

In sexual arousal, the brain sends signals via the nervous system and bloodstream to the spongy expandable cavernosae of the penis:

1. Components of the central nervous system release the chemical neurotransmitter messenger ACh that signals the cells of the endothelium to form nitric oxide (eNO) from L-arginine by the action of the eNOS.
2. In the vascular smooth muscle penis cavernosae, eNO signals the release of another enzyme sequence that helps to form cGMP (*cyclic guanosine monophosphate*).
3. cGMP is the actual vasodilator that relaxes the cavernosae smooth muscle, increasing blood inflow. (12)
4. As blood inflow rises in the cavernosae, the increased inflow and pressure cause shear stress on the endothelium that results in the additional release of eNOS and further maintenance of NO formation.
5. As blood fills the cavernosae, they expand, exerting pressure on the veins that lie between the *albuginea* and the *tunica*. This pressure constricts the veins, thus limiting blood outflow.
6. However, at the same time, there is also the formation and buildup of the enzyme phosphodiesterase type-5 (PDE5) that breaks down cGMP, causing reabsorption of the constituents, thus ending erection.

What Dr. L. Ignarro discovered was that if one has endothelium damage caused by health hazards such as atherosclerosis, or diabetes, but one can still form NO, albeit in insufficient amounts for satisfactory sexual "performance," then one can be helped by disabling the reabsorption enzyme PDE5. This led to the development of agents such as Viagra® (Sildenafil) that protect NO formation. These are aptly called *PDE5 inhibitors*. However, in the face of a seriously impaired endothelium, even PDE5 inhibitors may not work.

8.9 THE ROLE OF AGING IN ED

Americans are living longer now than they did just a few decades ago. According to the 2011 *CIA World Book*, average life expectancy in the United States was 78.37 years. Women live somewhat longer than men. There is little evidence of widespread loss of interest in sexuality in our "maturing" population. As we age, issues of sexuality for men and women diverge: while desire remains relatively high in older men, it can drop precipitously in most women in menopause.

Common myths make a compelling case for dismissing the lack of interest of seniors in lovemaking as there is still a residual attitude that sexuality as we reach the "golden years" is really not altogether proper. However, soaring sales of meds like Viagra® tell a different story: it's not all in the head, and it's not all just about age, but some of it is.

Seniors do face a challenge as the years pile up. There are anatomical changes in the cavernosal endothelium in men as they age and in the comparable clitoral cavernosae in postmenopausal women in whom decreased hormones of desire reduce both libido and the ability to maintain sexual intercourse comfortably.

ED is of great concern to many men especially as they age. A number of misconceptions cloud our understanding of the extent of ED in American men. For instance, a press release dated August 5, 2003, from the Harvard School of Public Health, titled "Prevalence of Erectile Dysfunction Increases With Age," tells us that fewer than 2% of the men in the study who reported that they had erection problems experienced them before the age of 40, and 4% had experienced problems between age 40 and 49. From age 50 upwards, the percentage of men reporting ED increased dramatically with 26% between the ages of 50 to 59, 40% aged 60 to 69 years and 61% for men older than 70 having experienced ED. (13)

The Harvard press release avers that "61 percent [of] men older than 70 [have] experienced ED," but it does not define "experienced." In fact, in a Massachusetts Male Aging Study (MMAS), it was shown that only about 15% of men in that age group were totally impotent, while less than 30% of them experienced "moderate" ED. Clearly, the manner of presenting data can give a different impression of the facts.

The MMAS study shows the likelihood that someone may experience either no dysfunction, minimal dysfunction, moderate or complete dysfunction. This is a more meaningful way to describe sexuality in populations of men as they age. In women, testosterone also is pretty much minimal by age 45, leading to loss of estrogen from which they derive it. Whereas in men, both free testosterone and free dihydrotestosterone remain relatively high well past that age. In fact, free dihydrotestosterone levels in men remain higher than free testosterone levels up to about age 70. (14, 15)

Hormonal issues notwithstanding, the evidence clearly shows that the NO/cGMP mechanism affects the response to sexual arousal in both men and women. Much has been published about that response in men, and the research on the role of that mechanism in women has been neglected. However, we know that there are age-related changes in the clitoris cavernosae like those in the penis cavernosae in aging men:

The *Journal of Urology* reported a strong link between increasing age and decreased clitoral cavernosal smooth muscle fibers. In the post-mortem tissue samples studied, not only did those decreases in cavernosal smooth muscle fibers correlate significantly with increase in age, but in the age group of 44 to 90 years, clitoral cavernosal fibrosis was found to be significantly greater in the presence of cardiovascular disease–related mortality compared with those without cardiovascular disease–related mortality. (16)

It's only a small jump from these data to the conclusion that women's physical arousal problems may also be linked to regularly consuming the SAD and to a sedentary lifestyle accelerating endothelial impairment just as happens in men. The authors did not pull their punches: *"Vascular risk factors may adversely affect the structure of clitoral cavernosal tissue."* In other words, it is impaired endothelium and thus, impaired NO/cGMP formation.

Aging has a significant adverse impact on sexual response both in men and in women, and medical authorities agree that it is due to progressive impairment of the endothelium and its ability to serve us NO when and where needed. Parenthetically, Sildenafil (Viagra®) increases clitoral and uterine blood flow in healthy postmenopausal women, even without any erotic stimulation. (17) The question remains, does NO production *ipso facto* decrease with age in men in parallel with declining erectile function?

8.9.1 Do We Just Run Out of Gas as We Age?

Contrary to common belief, testosterone, the hormone of desire, does not decrease much as we age, but NO production that fuels performance declines precipitously.

In 1996, a report in the journal *Hypertension* concluded that with age, eNO formation is impaired. This decline is detailed below in Figure 8.4.

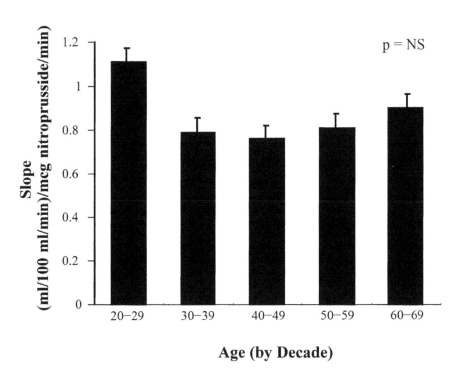

Age (by Decade)

FIGURE 8.2 Endothelium-dependent NO/cGMP) blood vessel relaxation decreases with age. [(18) Gerhard M, Roddy MA, Creager SJ, and MA Creager. 1996. Aging progressively impairs endothelium-dependent vasodilation in forearm resistance vessels of humans. *Hypertension*, Apr; 27(4): 849–853. DOI:10.1161/01.hyp.27.4.849.]

The investigators found that in people ranging in age from 19 to 90, NO/cGMP was progressively, and dramatically, impaired with increasing age. Furthermore, the decline is already evident by the fourth decade (age 30 to 39 years). (18) The fuel for performance declines in men just as they begin to produce a super testosterone hormone of desire, DHT.

Parenthetically, in addition to age, total cholesterol and low-density lipoprotein cholesterol were also predictors of NO/cGMP formation impairment. It seems that we have found diet and lifestyle ways of replicating the blunder in Dr. Furgott's lab.

The investigators concluded that age is the most significant predictor of NO/cGMP formation impairment, even in healthy persons. It stands to reason that oxidative stress lifestyle factors, including inactivity, damage our endothelium, thus causing our cardiovascular and health hazards to accumulate as we age.

Likewise, a clinical study published in the *European Journal of Preventive Cardiology* in 2013 found that flow-mediated dilation* (FMD) decreases significantly with increasing age in both genders up to 70 years for men and 80 for women.

In women, age-related decline in FMD was steepest after age 45; in men, there is a steady decline after age 30. Curiously, in men 80 years and older, FMD was higher than in men aged 50–79 years. We suspect a curious bias here: it may be that the men who survive to that age are endowed with a healthier cardiovascular system, reflected in less FMD impairment. (28)

8.10 ENDOTHELIUM DYSFUNCTION IS A FEATURE OF ED

According to a report published in the *Journal of Andrology*, the earliest detectable changes in vascular disease states associated with ED are abnormalities of the endothelium causing a loss in its normal homeostatic mechanisms that conventionally protect against disease-related processes. Considering the crucial role of the endothelium, it is not surprising that conditions that cause endothelial dysfunction, such as aging, diabetes, cardiovascular disease and hypercholesterolemia, are closely associated with ED. Normal penile erection requires coordinated arterial endothelium-dependent vasodilation, i.e., NO-dependent. (19)

8.11 ENTER FLAXSEED

Recapitulating the ACh/NO/cGMP pathway to sexual performance: the brain sends out ACh when we are sexually stimulated. It does not ordinarily have any problem doing that. ACh triggers NO formation by the endothelium of the blood vessel–like spongy cavernosae chambers of the penis. NO then causes the formation of the vessel-relaxing cGMP. If there is adequate NO formation, there will be adequate cGMP formation to cause and sustain erection. If NO formation is poor, type-5PDE will mop up what little there is of cGMP, and the result is little if any erection. The whole

---

* To measure FMD, the brachial artery is first bound to stop blood flow. Then the ligature is released and dilation is observed when blood flow is restored in the artery. The primary mediator of FMD is a release of NO by endothelial cells. (32)

cycle depends on NO, and the NO-donors in flaxseed and flax oil are an excellent way of supplying it.

There are a number of ways that flaxseed contributes to enhanced male performance.

8.11.1 FLAXSEED SUPPLIES L-ARGININE, THE SUBSTRATE FOR NO

First, flaxseed supplies L-arginine. A number of publications support supplementing L-arginine in treatment of ED. For instance, a meta-analysis published in the *Journal of Sexual Medicine* encompassed studies published up to April 2018 that evaluated the efficacy of arginine supplements identified from multiple databases such as Google Scholar, PubMed, Medline, Embase, Kiss, DBpia and Cochrane databases. The studies in the meta-analysis compared arginine supplements to placebo or no treatment, focusing only on patients with mild to moderate severity of ED, and presenting outcomes such as improvement rate, International Index of Erectile Function (IIEF) score and adverse effects.

The analysis demonstrated that arginine supplements with a dosage ranging from 1,500 to 5,000 mg/day significantly improved ED compared with placebo or no treatment. Arginine supplements also caused significant improvements in the IIEF subdomain scores of overall satisfaction, intercourse satisfaction, orgasmic function and erectile function, whereas the IIEF sexual desire scores remain unchanged. The adverse effect rate in the arginine-treated group was 8.3% and that in the placebo group was 2.3%, none of which were severe. (20)

A clinical study published in the journal *Andrologia* examined the effects of L-arginine supplementation in medical (pharmacological) treatment of ED: the study compared the clinical efficacy of daily use of L-arginine, tadalafil, and combined L-arginine with tadalafil (Cialis), in the treatment of elderly patients with erectile dysfunction. Daily oral L-arginine (5 grams), or tadalafil (5 mg), or L-arginine (5 grams) combined with tadalafil (5 mg), or placebo were taken for 6 weeks in each group of patients, respectively.

Patients were assessed before and after treatments using the Sexual Health Inventory for Men (SHIM) questionnaire and total serum testosterone. The means of Q1–5, total scores of SHIM and total testosterone in L-arginine, tadalafil and combined L-arginine with tadalafil groups were significantly higher after treatments. Combined L-arginine with tadalafil group had the highest SHIM scores and levels of total tetosterone.

The investigators concluded that combining daily L-arginine with tadalafil therapy for elderly male ED patients could significantly increase SHIM scores and levels of total testosterone compared to L-arginine or tadalafil alone. (21) In other words, increasing NO bioavailability by L-arginine supplementation enhances the effects of tadalafil, a medical/pharmacological PDE5 inhibitor.

8.11.2 ROS JEOPARDIZE ERECTILE FUNCTION

The antioxidant properties of flaxseed and flax oil, in addition to these substances being NO-donors, cannot be overemphasized insofar as it has been shown that oxidative stress is a feature in both cardiovascular diseases (CVD) and ED involving the overproduction of ROS, in particular, superoxide ($O_2^{\bullet-}$) and hydrogen peroxide (H_2O_2). (22)

Furthermore, in an article titled the "Role of Oxidative Stress in the Pathophysiological Mechanism of Erectile Dysfunction," published in the *Journal of Andrology*, the investigators report that increased production of ROS is associated with decreased normal erectile response, primarily because of reduced NO concentrations. Increased production of ROS in diseases such as diabetes and hypertension might be an important cause of an increased risk of ED. (23)

8.11.3 FLAXSEED SUPPLIES THE ANTIOXIDANT OMEGA-3 FATTY ACIDS PROMOTING eNO FORMATION

There are no conventional medical publications that address the potential role of cyanogenic glycosides in connection with ED. But flax supplies omega-3 fatty acids. and a number of publications report that these enhance sexual function by various means.

For instance, it has been well established that oxidative stress and inflammation disrupt NO production directly or by, among other things, increasing resistance to insulin. This action is a documented contribution to determinants of vascular diseases, including ED. Men with ED have decreased vascular NO, as well as decreased circulating and cellular antioxidants. Also, oxidative stress and inflammatory markers are increased in men with ED, and these increase with age.

Potent antioxidants or high doses of weaker antioxidants increase vascular NO and improve vascular and erectile function. Antioxidants may be particularly important in men with ED who smoke, are obese or have diabetes.

It is reported in the *International Journal of Impotence Research* that omega-3 fatty acids reduce inflammatory markers, decrease cardiac death and increase endothelial NO production, and are therefore critical for men with ED who are under age 60 years and/or have diabetes, hypertension or coronary artery disease and are at increased risk of serious or even fatal cardiac events. (24)

The link between ED and cardiovascular disease is now so well-known that a subset of the authors of the aforementioned report called that link "the canary in the coal mine" in a study published in the *American Journal of Cardio*logy. (25)

The supplementation of omega-3 fatty acids from flaxseed or flax oil in ED may be particularly cogent since it was reported in a study published in the journal *Lipids in Health and Disease* that fatty acid metabolism is "disturbed" in ED. The study concerned ED in type 2 diabetes patients because vasculogenic erectile dysfunction is considered a common complication in that population.

The study aimed to determine whether changes in fatty acid classes measured in erythrocytes are associated with increased risk of diabetic vasculogenic erectile dysfunction (VED) along with related risk factors. The investigators assessed erythrocyte (red blood cell) fatty acids composition, lipid peroxidation parameters and inflammatory cytokines in type 2 diabetes patients with VED compared to that in healthy volunteers.

It was found that diabetic patients had significantly lower indices of Δ6-desaturase and elongase activities compared to the other studied groups. The same group of participants displayed lower erythrocyte levels of dihomo-γ-linolenic acid precursor of the messenger molecule PGE1 mainly involved in promoting erection. Moreover, absolute saturated fatty acids (SFA)s concentration and HOMA-IR levels were higher in type 2 diabetes patients with VED when compared to controls, and associated with impaired NO concentration.

The results showed that IL-6 and TNF-α were significantly increased and positively correlated with malondialdehyde level (MDA, a marker of oxidative stress) only in type 2 diabetes people with VED, suggesting a decrease in the relative availability of vasodilator mediators and activation of vasoconstrictors release.

The investigators concluded that the "deranged" fatty acids metabolism constitutes a marker of vasculogenic erectile dysfunction in progress, or at least an indicator of increased risk within men with type 2 diabetes. (26)

- *Δ6-desaturase, or delta-6-desaturase enzyme, is one of two rate limiting enzymes that convert the polyunsaturated fatty acid (PUFA) precursors α-linolenic (omega-3) and linoleic acid (omega-6) to their respective metabolites. Changes in the delta-6-desaturase enzyme activity alter fatty acid profiles and are associated with metabolic and inflammatory diseases including cardiovascular disease and type 2 diabetes.*
- *Elongase is a generic term for an enzyme that catalyzes carbon chain extension of an organic molecule, especially a fatty acid. Elongases play a variety of roles in mammalian organisms, accounting for changes in tissue function and lipid regulation.*
- *Dihomo-γ-linolenic acid is an omega-6 PUFA.*
- *HOMA-IR, homeostatic model assessment for insulin resistance is an index of insulin resistance.*
- *PGE1 is a smooth muscle relaxant and is used as a vasodilator medication in the management of erectile dysfunction and ductus arteriosus in neonates.*
- *IL-6 is a cytokine with broad-ranging effects in the immune response. One of the roles of IL-6 is to support immunocompetence, the ability of a host to respond to infections.*
- *TNF-α: Tumor necrosis factor alpha is an inflammatory cytokine produced by macrophages/monocytes during acute inflammation.*

Finally, in a meta-analysis published in the *Iranian Journal of Basic Medical Sciences*, the investigators report that the main constituents of flaxseed include lipids, proteins, lignans, fibers and minerals, and flaxseed contains antioxidants such as tocopherols, beta-carotene, cysteine and methionine, which result in a decrease in blood pressure; reduced risk of heart disease, as well as of hepatic and neurological disorders; and increased insulin sensitivity, and because flaxseed is commonly used for its antidiabetic and anticancer activities, benefiting also cardiovascular, gastrointestinal, hepatic, urological and reproductive disorders; therefore, it is recognized as a medical plant. (27)

8.12 SUMMARY

In most clinical cases, ED is not due to emotional inhibitions or lack of desire but to organic dysfunction preventing sexual stimulation from leading to increased blood flow to the genitals in both men and women. Recent research has shown that this deficit commonly results from impaired NO formation in the endothelium thought to be damaged by oxidative stress. Flaxseed supplies L-arginine, the substrate for NO; and cyanogenic glycosides, a NO-donor; and the omega-3 fatty acids that supply antioxidants to combat further free radical damage.

8.13 REFERENCES

1. Irwig MS, and S Kolukula. 2012. Persistent sexual side effects of Finasteride for male pattern hair loss. *Journal of Sex Medicine*, 8(6): 1747–1753. DOI:10.1111/j.1743-6109.2011.02255.x.
2. Wagner G, and R Green. 1972. Testosterone secretion and metabolism in male senescence. *Journal of Clinical Endocrinology*, Apr; 34(4): 730–735. DOI:10.1210/jcem-34-4-730.
3. Vermeulen A, Rubens R, and L Verdonck. 1972. Testosterone secretion and metabolism in male senescence. *Journal of Clinical Endocrinology*, Apr; 34(4): 730–735. DOI:10.1210/jcem-34-4-730.
4. Furchgott RF, and JV Zawadzki. 1980. The obligatory role of endothelial cells in the relaxation of arterial smooth muscle by acetylcholine. *Nature*, Nov 27; 288(5789): 373–376. DOI:10.1038/288373a0.
5. Moncada S, and A Higgs. 1993. The L-arginine-nitric oxide pathway. *NEJM*, Dec 30; 329(27): 2002–2012. DOI:10.1056/NEJM199312303292706.
6. Oberleithner H, Peters W, Kusche-Vihrog K, Korte S, Schillers S, Kliche K, and K Oberleithner. 2011. Salt overload damages the glycocalyx sodium barrier of vascular endothelium. *Pflugers Archives*, Oct; 462(4): 519–528. DOI:10.1007/s00424-011-0999-1.
7. Nieuwdorp M, van Haeften TW, Gouverneur MCLG, Mooij HL, van Lieshout MHP, Levi M, Meijers JCM, Holleman F, Hoekstra JBL, Vink H, Kastelein JJP, and ESG Stroes. 2006. Loss of endothelial glycocalyx during acute hyperglycemia coincides with endothelial dysfunction and coagulation activation in vivo. *Diabetes*, Feb; 55(2): 480–486. DOI:10.2337/diabetes.55.02.06.db05-1103.
8. Ikonomidis I, Voumvourakis A, Makavos G, Triantafyllidi H, Pavlidis G, Katogiannis K, Benas D, Vlastos D, Trivilou P, Varoudi M, Parissi J, Lliodromitis E, and J Lekakis. 2018. Association of impaired endothelial glycocalyx with arterial stiffness, coronary microcirculatory dysfunction, and abnormal myocradial deformation in untreated hypertensives. *Journal of Clinical Hypertension*, 20: 672–679. DOI:10.1111/jch.13236.
9. Harding IC, Mitra R, Mensah SA, Herman IM, and EE Ebong. 2018. Pro-atherosclerotic disturbed flow disrupts caveolin-1 expression, localization, and function via glycocalyx degradation. *Journal of Translational Medicine*, Dec 18; 16(364). DOI:10.1186/s12967-018-1721-2.
10. Yamaoka-Tojoab M. 2020. Endothelial glycocalyx damage as a systemic inflammatory microvascular endotheliopathy in COVID-19. *Biomedical Journal*, Oct; 43(5): 399–413. DOI:10.1016/j.bj.2020.08.007.
11. Bartosch AMW, Mathews R, and JM Tarbell. 2017. Endothelial glycocalyx-mediated nitric oxide production in response to selective AFM pulling. *Biophysics Journal*, Jul 11; 113(1): 101–108. DOI:10.1016/j.bpj.2017.05.033.
12. Murphy RA, and JS Walker. 1998. Inhibitory mechanisms for cross-bridge cycling: The nitric oxide-cGMP signal transduction pathway in smooth muscle relaxation. *Acta Physiologica Scandinavica*, 164: 373–380.

13. https://archive.sph.harvard.edu/press-releases/archives/2003-releases/press08052003.html.
14. Feldman HA, Goldstein I, Hatzichristou DG, Krane RJ, and JB McKinlay. 1994. Impotence and its medical and psychosocial correlates: Results of the Massachusetts Male Aging Study. *Journal of Urology*, 151: 54–61.
15. Stárka L, Pospíšilová H, and M Hill. 2009. Free testosterone and free dihydrotestosterone throughout the life span of men. *Journal of Steroid Biochemistry and Molecular Biology*, 116(1–2): 118–120. DOI:10.1016/j.jsbmb.2009.05.008.
16. Tarcan T, Park K, Goldstein I, Maio G, Fassina A, Krane RJ, and KM Azadzoi. 1999. Histomorphometric analysis of age-related structural changes in human clitoral cavernosal tissue. *Journal of Urology*, Mar; 161: 940–944. PMID: 10022730.
17. Alatas E, and AB Yagci. 2004. The effect of Sildenafil citrate on uterine and clitoral arterial blood flow in postmenopausal women. *Medscap General Medicine*, 13(6): 51. PMCID: PMC1480594.
18. Gerhard M, Roddy MA, Creager SJ, and MA Creager. 1996. Aging progressively impairs endothelium-dependent vasodilation in forearm resistance vessels of humans. *Hypertension*, Apr; 27(4): 849–853. DOI:10.1161/01.hyp.27.4.849.
19. Bivalacqua TJ, Usta MF, Champion HC, Kadowitz PJ, and WJG Hellstrom. 2003. Endothelial dysfunction in erectile dysfunction: Role of the endothelium in erectile physiology and disease. *Journal of Andrology*, Nov–Dec; 24(S6): S17–S37. DOI:10.1002/j.1939-4640.2003.tb02743.x.
20. Rhim HC, Kim MS, Park Y-J, Suk Choi WS, Park HK, Kim HG, Kim A, and SH Paick. 2019. The potential role of arginine supplements on erectile dysfunction: A systemic review and meta-analysis. *Journal of Sexual Medicine*, Feb; 16(2): 223–234. DOI:10.1016/j.jsxm.2018.12.002.
21. El-Hamd MA, and EM Hegaz. 2020. Comparison of the clinical efficacy of daily use of L-arginine, tadalafil and combined L-arginine with tadalafil in the treatment of elderly patients with erectile dysfunction. *Andrologia*, Aug; 52(7): e13640. DOI:10.1111/and.13640.
22. Jeremy JY, Jones RA, Koupparis AJ, Hotston M, Persad R, Angelini GD, and N Shukla. 2006. Reactive oxygen species and erectile dysfunction: Possible role of NADPH oxidase. *International Journal of Impotence Research*, Oct 16; 19: 265–280. DOI:10.1038/sj.ijir.3901523.
23. Agarwal A, Nandipati KC, Sharma RK, Zippe CD, and R Raina. 2006. Role of oxidative stress in the pathophysiological mechanism of erectile dysfunction. *Journal of Andrology*, May–June; 27(3): 335–347. DOI:10.2164/jandrol.05136.
24. Meldrum DR, Gambone JC, Morris MA, Esposito K, Giugliano D, and LJ Ignarro. 2011. Lifestyle and metabolic approaches to maximizing erectile and vascular health. *International Journal of Impotence Research*, Nov 10; 24: 61–68. DOI:10.1038/19ijir.2011.51.
25. Meldrum DR, Gambone JC, Morris M, Meldrum DAN, Esposito K, and LJ Ignarro. 2011. The link between erectile and cardiovascular health: The canary in the coal mine. *American Journal of Cardiology*, Aug 15; 108(4): 599–606. DOI:10.1016/j.amjcard.2011.03.093.
26. Ben Khedher MR, Bouhajja H, Ahmed SH, Abid M, Jamoussi K, and M Hammami. 2017. Role of disturbed fatty acids metabolism in the pathophysiology of diabetic erectile dysfunction. *Lipids in Health and Disease*, 16: 241. DOI:10.1186/s12944-017-0637-9.
27. Ebrahimi B, Nazmara Z, Hassanzadeh N, Yarahmadi A, Ghaffari N, Hassani F, Liaghat A, Noori L, and G Hassanzadeh. 2012. Biomedical features of flaxseed against different pathologic situations: A narrative review. *Iranian Journal of Basic Medical Sciences*, May; 24(5): 551–560. DOI:10.22038/ijbms.2021.49821.11378.

28. Skaug E-A, Aspenes ST, Oldervoll L, Mørkedal B, Vatten L, Wisløff U, and O Ellingsen. 2013. Age and gender differences of endothelial function in 4739 healthy adults: The HUNT3 fitness study. *European Journal of Preventive Cardiology*, Aug; 20(4): 531–540. DOI:10.1177/2047487312444234.+
29. Ustuner ET. 2013. Cause of androgenic alopecia: Crux of the matter. *Plastic and Reconstructive Surgery Global Open*, Oct; 7: e64. DOI:10.1097/GOX.0000000000000005.
30. Rodríguez-García C, Sánchez-Quesada C, Toledo E, Delgado-Rodríguez M, and JJ Gaforio. 2019. Naturally lignan-rich foods: A dietary tool for health promotion? *Molecules*, Mar; 24(5): 917. DOI:10.3390/molecules24050917.
31. Whittaker J, and K Wu. 2021. Low-fat diets and testosterone in men: Systematic review and meta-analysis of intervention studies. *Journal of Steroid Biochemistry and Molecular Biology*. Jun; 210: 105878. DOI:10.1016/j.jsbmb.2021.105878.
32. Kelm M. 2002. Flow-mediated dilatation in human circulation: Diagnostic and therapeutic aspects. *American Journal of Physiology*, Jan; 282(1): H1–H5. DOI:10.1152/ajpheart.2002.282.1.H1.

9 Omega-3 PUFA and L-Arginine for Longer Life Span with a Longer Health Span

9.1 ONE WAY TO LONGER LIFE IS TO PREVENT SHORTENING IT

The first eight chapters of this book examined the basic benefits of flaxseed constituents, i.e., L-arginine, omega-3 polyunsaturated fatty acids (PUFAs) and cyanogenic glycosides. What this examination revealed at the level of the tissues and organs is that these constituents seem to bestow their benefits principally on blood vessels and the heart by supporting endothelial (and endocardial) function by their antioxidant action and by setting the stage, as it were, for enhancing nitric oxide (NO) formation.

We focused mainly on omega-3 PUFAs because they are far more plentiful in flaxseed and in flax oil than omega-6s. But keep in mind that flaxseed contains both omega-3 and omega-6 fatty acids, both of which promote good health. In fact, omega-6 PUFAs were shown to reduce the risk of coronary heart disease. (1) So both are beneficial, but it is not the ratio that really counts because you can have a low 6:3 ratio and in the end still wind up with low absolute levels of omega-3 in the tissues. What matters is the amount of omega-3s that one gets, not so much the ratio.

Flaxseed oil is about 50% to 60% omega-3 fatty acids, mainly alpha-linolenic acid (ALA). That is more than is contained in fish oil. The omega-6 to omega-3 PUFAs ratio is 1:4, which is ideal. Some researchers think flaxseed oil might have some of the same benefits as fish oil. But the body is not very efficient at converting ALA into EPA and DHA. The ALA that is so abundant in flaxseed oil is not readily converted by the body into EPA and DHA. So, in the first eight chapters, we described prevention and treatment of cardiovascular and related risk factors with these nutrients. But here, we'll focus also on forestalling catastrophe.

Omega-3 PUFAs prevent life span from being shortened because one pathway to longevity is, to put it bluntly, avoiding death from cardiovascular disease. As WS Harris put it in the title of his 2016 publication in the journal *Atherosclerosis*, "[low levels of] RBC omega-3 predicts risk for death." (2)

Think about this: according to the Centers for Disease Control and Prevention, there are four major cardiovascular disease risk factors: high blood pressure, unhealthy blood cholesterol levels, diabetes mellitus and obesity. (3) There are others, of course, including smoking, abusing alcohol and/or drugs, heredity and so on, but these are said to be the major ones.

According to a report recently published in the *American Journal of Clinical Nutrition* in 2021, fatty acids concentration was measured in red blood cells from a cohort followed for 11 years. It was found that the information conveyed by tests on the concentrations of fatty acids obtained from red blood cells was as useful as the information conveyed by tests of lipid levels, blood pressure, smoking and diabetic status in predicting total mortality. (4) In that study, the investigators used levels of erythrocyte fatty acids ("fingerprint") to predict risk of all-cause mortality in the Framingham Offspring Cohort. Their report provides some additional gems:

The fatty acids most clearly associated with reduced risk for cardiovascular disease (CVD) and for total mortality (i.e., death from any cause) are the omega-3 PUFAs, eicosapentaenoic (EPA) (20: 5n–3) and docosahexaenoic (DHA) (22: 6n–3).

Likewise, a report published in the journal *Circulation: Cardiovascular Quality and Outcomes* in 2010, was titled "Blood Eicosapentaenoic and Docosahexaenoic Acids Predict All-Cause Mortality in Patients with Stable Coronary Heart Disease: The Heart and Soul Study." (5)

In yet another study, published in the journal *Annals of Internal Medicine*, in 2013, the investigators send the very clear message that "higher circulating individual and total ω3-PUFA levels are associated with lower total mortality, especially CHD death, in older adults." (6)

A report published in the *Journal of Clinical Lipidology* in 2018 describes a study where participants in the Framingham Offspring Cohort were followed for a median of 7.3 years (i.e., between ages ~66 and 73 y). It was found that the baseline red blood cell (erythrocytes) EPA + DHA content (the Omega-3 Index) was significantly inversely associated with risk for death from all causes. Individuals in the highest quintile were 33% less likely to succumb during the follow-up years compared with those in the lowest quintile. (7)

The investigators reported that "*a higher omega-3 index was associated with reduced risk of both CVD and all-cause mortality.*" The Omega Index, developed by Drs. WS Harris and C. Von Schacky in 2004 is described in greater detail in a later section of this chapter. (27) Similar findings were observed in the Women's Health Initiative Memory Study: the purpose of the prospective cohort study, also published in the *Journal of Clinical Lipidology*, albeit earlier, in 2017, was to determine the associations between red blood cells (RBC) PUFA levels and risk for death. The study centered on men and women aged 65 to 80 years who participated in the Women's Health Initiative Memory Study (enrollment began in 1996). The primary "outcome" was total mortality through August 2014.

It was found that after a median of 14.9 years of follow-up, 1,851 women (28.5%) had died. RBC levels of EPA and DHA were significantly higher in the survivors.

In the fully adjusted models, the *hazard ratios*[*] (99% confidence intervals) for mortality associated with 1 standard deviation PUFA increase for total mortality

---

[*] The hazard ratio is an estimate of the ratio of the hazard rate in a treatment group versus that in a control group.

were 0.92 (0.85, 0.98) for the Omega-3 Index, 0.89 (0.82, 0.96) for EPA, 0.93 (0.87, 1.0) for DHA and 0.76 (0.64, 0.90) for the PUFA factor score. There was no significant specific differentiation between ALA, arachidonic acid or linoleic acid with total mortality. The investigators concluded that higher RBC levels of marine omega-3 PUFAs predicted reduced risk for all-cause mortality. (8)

A study conducted in Germany, published in the journal *Atherosclerosis*, in 2016, reported that EPA and DHA were associated with reduced mortality in patients referred for coronary angiography in the Ludwigshafen Risk and Cardiovascular Health Study, independent of other risk factors, with the association of EPA with mortality being nonlinear. (9)

The message is unambiguous: omega-3 fatty acids promote health and in fact, forestall death from cardiovascular disease. The good news: omega-3 fatty acids are plentiful in flaxseed.

9.2 HOW CAN WE TELL WHETHER PEOPLE WHO CONSUME FLAXSEED OR FLAX OIL AGE MORE SLOWLY, LIVE LONGER?

Most of our cells have a nucleus that contains chromosomes. The chromosomes end in telomeres, special structures that provide protection from enzymatic end-degradation and maintain chromosomal and genomic stability. For this reason, adequate telomere structure (including the presence of telomere-binding proteins) remains the key to avoiding cellular dysfunction.

With each cell replication, telomeres shorten. There is a consensus that not only is their length reduced by aging as cells divide to replicate but also that the process can be accelerated by *metabolic stress*, among other factors, and that shorter telomeres can impair health and longevity. Thus, slowing telomere shortening or, at least, not accelerating the process, is to our advantage in preserving our natural life span.

You may recall the Greek myth of the three *Fates* who control the mother thread of life from birth to death. Clotho spun the thread of life, Lachesis measured the thread allotted to each person and Atropos was the cutter of the thread, choosing the moment of each person's passing. You can substitute "metabolic stress" for Atropos, and "telomeres" for the "thread of life."

9.2.1 OMEGA-3S CONCENTRATION AFFECTS CELL AGING VIA TELOMERE LENGTH

Shorter telomeres have been associated with oxidative stress, poor health behaviors—so-called lifestyle factors—age-related diseases, and early mortality. Telomere length is regulated by the enzyme *telomerase* and is linked to exposure to proinflammatory cytokines and oxidative stress.

In a study titled "Omega-3 Fatty Acids, Oxidative Stress, and Leukocyte Telomere Length: A Randomized Controlled Trial," published in the journal *Brain, Behavior and Immunity*, in 2013, omega-3 PUFA supplementation was found to lower the concentration of serum proinflammatory cytokines. The study aimed to determine whether omega-3 PUFA supplementation also affected leukocyte telomere length, telomerase and oxidative stress.

The study was conducted on healthy sedentary overweight middle-aged and older adults who received (1) 2.5 g/day omega-3 PUFAs, (2) 1.25 g/day omega-3 PUFAs or (3) placebo capsules that mirrored the proportions of fatty acids in the typical American diet.

It was found that the supplementation significantly lowered oxidative stress. Changes in the omega-6/omega-3 PUFA plasma ratios reflected in telomere length significantly increased with decreasing ratios. A decreasing omega-6 to omega-3 ratio means that there are more omega-3s and that the increase in omega-3s (relative to omega-6s) is associated with longer telomere length.

The investigators concluded that lower omega-6/omega-3 PUFA ratios can beneficially impact cell aging. And, furthermore, "The triad of inflammation, oxidative stress, and immune cell aging represents important pre-disease mechanisms that may be ameliorated through nutritional interventions." (10)

Myocardial "remodeling" is a continuum of changes in the structure and function of the myocardium. That commonly occurs as a result of aging or of pathological processes. Adverse myocardial remodeling is associated with poor patient outcomes in the context of ischemic heart disease and/or myocardial infarction, cardiac hypertrophy and cardiomyopathic disease states. (11)

Remodeling of myocardial cell membranes, then, is an aspect of advanced age. Mitochondrial function, crucial to sustaining energy production and management of myocardial metabolism, is impacted by age-dependent remodeling and ultimately exhibits a diminished threshold for excess Ca^{2+} buffering during events that stimulate increased myocardial Ca^{2+}, such as augmented cardiac work, oxidative stress or post-ischemic reflow.

In a study published in the journal *Experimental Gerontology*, in 2005, it was reported that a diet rich in omega-3 PUFA reverses the age-associated membrane omega-6:omega-3 PUFA imbalance, and dysfunctional Ca^{2+} metabolism, facilitating increased efficiency of mitochondrial energy production and improved tolerance of ischemia and reperfusion. (12)

9.2.2 Omega-3 PUFAs Slow Aging by Lowering Mitochondria Free Radical "Emissions"

We derive energy by combining food-derived "fuel" with oxygen. We call this "oxidative metabolism," and the structures in our cells largely responsible for this process are the mitochondria. Although we are exposed to a panoply of environmentally produced oxygen free radicals, one by-product of oxidative metabolism is a large outpouring of free radicals. These combine with other substances in our body to form ROS.

A prominent theory of aging is the Harman theory, i.e., that aging is due, in large part, to the corrosive action of ROS on DNA, i.e. metabolic stress. (26) Omega-3 polyunsaturated fatty acids (omega-3 PUFA) are known anti-inflammatory antioxidants that may be beneficial in the treatment of loss of muscle tissue as a natural part of the aging process (sarcopenia). A clinical study published in the journal *Aging* in 20127 aimed to determine the effects of omega-3 PUFA on muscle mitochondrial physiology and protein metabolism in older adults.

Young men (18–35 years) and older men (65–85 years) and women were studied at baseline. Older adults were then studied again following 3.9g/day of omega-3 PUFA supplementation for 16 weeks. Muscle biopsies were used to evaluate respiratory capacity (high-resolution respirometry) and oxidant emissions (spectrofluorometry) in isolated mitochondria. It was found that maximal respiration was significantly lower in older compared to young participants. Omega-3 PUFA supplements significantly reduced oxidant emissions.

Following omega-3 PUFA supplementation, mixed muscle, mitochondrial and sarcoplasmic protein synthesis rates were increased in older adults before exercise. Omega-3 PUFA increased post-exercise mitochondrial and myofibrillar protein synthesis in older adults.

The investigators concluded that omega-3 PUFA supplements reduce mitochondrial oxidant emissions, increase postabsorptive muscle protein synthesis and enhance anabolic responses to exercise in older adults. In other words, omega-3 PUFA supplementation reduced "mitochondrial oxidant emission" without adversely affecting metabolism. (13) Only antioxidant action could have accomplished that.

An experimental animal-model (mice) study published in the journal *Prostaglandins, Leukotrienes and Essential Fatty Acids*, in 2015, aimed to determine the effect of orally administered omega-3 (PUFA) on mitochondrial function and processing of the amyloid precursor protein in brains of young (3 months old) and aged (24 months old) Naval Medical Research Institute (NMRI)-mice.

The neuroprotective properties of 1.6 mL/kg p.o. of fish oil were assessed *ex vivo* after 21 days in dissociated brain cells and isolated mitochondria and it was found that DHA levels were significantly lower in the blood and brains of aged mice, which were not compensated by fish oil administration. Isolated dissociated brain cells and mitochondria from aged mice showed significantly lower adenosine triphosphate (ATP) levels and reduced activity of complexes I+II and IV of the mitochondrial respiration system, respectively. However, fish oil restored the age-related decrease in respiration and improved ATP production.

The investigators concluded that their findings reveal new mechanisms underlying the neuroprotective actions of omega-3 PUFA and identified fish oil as a promising nutraceutical to delay age-related mitochondrial dysfunction in the brain. (14) So, aging is not simply a musculoskeletal issue; it also entails cognitive function.

To wit: In a review titled "Omega-3 Fatty Acids and Brain Resistance to Ageing and Stress: Body of Evidence and Possible Mechanisms," published in the journal *Ageing Research Reviews* in 2013, the authors assert,

> The increasing life expectancy in the populations of rich countries raises the pressing question of how the elderly can maintain their cognitive function. Cognitive decline is characterised by the loss of short-term memory due to a progressive impairment of the underlying brain cell processes. Age-related brain damage has many causes, some of which may be influenced by diet. An optimal diet may therefore be a practical

way of delaying the onset of age-related cognitive decline. Nutritional investigations indicate that the ω-3 poyunsaturated fatty acid (PUFA) content of western diets is too low to provide the brain with an optimal supply of docosahexaenoic acid (DHA), the main ω-3 PUFA in cell membranes. Insufficient brain DHA has been associated with memory impairment, emotional disturbances and altered brain processes in rodents. Human studies suggest that an adequate dietary intake of ω-3 PUFA can slow the age-related cognitive decline and may also protect against the risk of senile dementia. However, despite the many studies in this domain, the beneficial impact of ω-3 PUFA on brain function has only recently been linked to specific mechanisms. This review examines the hypothesis that an optimal brain DHA status, conferred by an adequate ω-3 PUFA intake, limits age-related brain damage by optimizing endogenous brain repair mechanisms. Our analysis of the abundant literature indicates that an adequate amount of DHA in the brain may limit the impact of stress, an important age-aggravating factor, and influences the neuronal and astroglial functions that govern and protect synaptic transmission. This transmission, particularly glutamatergic neurotransmission in the hippocampus, underlies memory formation. The brain DHA status also influences neurogenesis, nested in the hippocampus, which helps maintain cognitive function throughout life. Although there are still gaps in our knowledge of the way ω-3 PUFA act, the mechanistic studies reviewed here indicate that ω-3 PUFA may be a promising tool for preventing age-related brain deterioration. (15) With permission.

Their review aims to determine whether an optimal brain DHA status derived from an adequate omega-3 PUFA intake, limits age-related brain damage by optimizing endogenous brain repair mechanisms. Based on their analysis, the authors conclude that an adequate amount of DHA in the brain may limit the impact of age-aggravating stress, influencing brain cell functions that govern and protect synaptic transmission. They concluded that omega-3 PUFA may be helpful in preventing age-related brain deterioration. (15)

9.2.3 Speaking of Cognitive Aging

There is considerable evidence that cognitive decline results not only from changes in brain health but also depends on nutritional status. Decline in the ability to think and reason abstractly and solve problems, i.e., "fluid intelligence," is one of the most debilitating aspects of cognitive aging. That decline has been linked to omega-3 PUFA deficiency. However, it is not known whether this phenomenon results from specific omega-3 PUFAs acting on particular aspects of brain function.

The aim of a clinical study published in the journal *Nutritional Neuroscience* (an *International Journal on Nutrition, Diet and Nervous System*), in 2018, was to determine whether omega-3 PUFAs influence fluid intelligence by supporting specific neural structures. The investigators measured six plasma phospholipid omega-3 PUFAs, fluid intelligence, and regional gray matter volume in the frontal and parietal cortices in 100 cognitively intact older adults (65–75 years old).

It was found that one pattern of omega-3 PUFAs, consisting of ALA, stearidonic acid and eicosatrienoic acid, was linked to fluid intelligence, and that total gray matter volume of the left frontoparietal cortex fully mediated the relationship between this omega-3 PUFA pattern and fluid intelligence.

The investigators concluded that fluid intelligence may be optimally supported by specific omega-3 PUFAs through the preservation of frontoparietal cortex gray matter structure in cognitively intact older adults. This report provides novel evidence for the anti-aging benefits of particular omega-3 PUFA patterns on fluid intelligence and underlying gray matter structure. (16)

9.3 CRITERIA FOR OMEGA-3 SUFFICIENCY: THE OMEGA-3 INDEX

Despite the evident need for assessing individual body concentrations of beneficial fatty acids, there is no simple home-testing means for doing so currently available to the typical consumer. Home measurement kits are available at pharmacies to measure blood pressure, arterial blood O_2 concentration, blood glucose and even blood lipids. In fact, there are few guidelines as to what criteria one might use to establish healthy vs. deficiency levels. So, how can the average individual who wishes to attain beneficial levels of omega-3s via diet or supplements know if s/he is successful? That is now changing.

A number of commercial laboratories provide "home test" kits that evaluate a small finger prick sample of blood for fatty acids composition and return a report to the purchaser with omega-3 concentration, the Omega Index. For instance, there are the following:

Omegaquant
5009 W. 12th Street, Suite 8
Sioux Falls, SD 57106
Phone: 1-605-271-6917
Toll-free: 1-800-949-0632
Fax: 1-800-526-9873
Email: info@omegaquant.com
Website: https://omegaquant.com/what-is-the-omega-3-index/ (accessed 1/12/22)

If one contacts them, they will send the customer a test kit to be returned to them with a drop of blood as instructed. They will then return a report indicating the Omega Index, a percentage value. Parenthetically, the laboratory procedure for determining the ratio of these fatty acids consists of determining their concentration in red blood cells. (17) Omegaquant also supplies the following information about cardiovascular "risk zones":

- High risk   = less than 4%
- Intermediate risk = 4% to 8%
- Low risk   = more than 8%

The Omega-3 Index as a risk factor for heart disease was first put forth in 2004 in the journal *Preventive Medicine* by Dr. WS Harris, who co-invented the Omega-3 Index test. It provides a percentage which is a measure of the amount of omega-3 fatty acids, eicosapentaenoic acid (EPA) and docosahexaenoic acid (DHA) in one's red blood cell membranes. An Omega-3 Index of 8% or higher is ideal, the lowest risk zone. If one's Omega-3 Index is in the optimal range, the omega-6 to omega-3 ratio should also be OK—it's all about the denominator. However, most people hover around 5% to 6% or less. And unfortunately in the United States, many people are at 4% or below—the highest risk zone.

As noted previously, in 2008, WS Harris published a report in the *American Journal of Clinical Nutrition*, which points out that

> Because blood concentrations of n-3 (or omega-3) fatty acids (FAs) (eicosapentaenoic and docosahexaenoic acids) are a strong reflection of dietary intake, it is proposed that a n-3 FA biomarker, the omega-3 index (erythrocyte eicosapentaenoic acid plus docosahexaenoic acid), be considered as a potential risk factor for coronary heart disease mortality, especially sudden cardiac death. The omega-3 index fulfills many of the requirements for a risk factor including consistent epidemiologic evidence, a plausible mechanism of action, a reproducible assay, independence from classic risk factors, modifiability, and, most important, the demonstration that raising levels will reduce risk for cardiac events. Measuring membrane concentrations of n-3 FAs is a rational approach to biostatus assessment as these FAs appear to exert their beneficial metabolic effects because of their actions in membranes. They alter membrane physical characteristics and the activity of membrane-bound proteins, and, once released by intracellular phospholipases from membrane stores, they can interact with ion channels, be converted into a wide variety of bioactive eicosanoids, and serve as ligands for several nuclear transcription factors, thereby altering gene expression. The omega-3 index compares very favorably with other risk factors for sudden cardiac death. Proposed omega-3 index risk zones are (in percentages of erythrocyte FAs): high risk, <4%; intermediate risk, 4–8%; and low risk, >8%. Before assessment of n-3 FA biostatus can be used in routine clinical evaluation of patients, standardized laboratory methods and quality control materials must become available. (18) With permission.

There is a compelling need for routine evaluation of blood concentrations of beneficial fatty acids in light of the fact that they may be as telling as the panoply of other routine blood tests currently in vogue. There is however a recent delineation of criteria and targets for optimal omega-3 concentrations. It was published in 2021 in the journal *BMJ Open*, in a report titled "Mean Serum LC Omega-3 Fatty Acid Concentrations (% of Total Fatty Acids) by Age Group in NHANES 2011–2012." You can access it at https://bmjopen.bmj.com/content/11/5/e043301.

Go to the PDF version, and you will see their second table: "*Comparisons are *children 3–19 years vs adults 20+ years, †early childhood and middle childhood vs adolescents, and ‡adults vs seniors. Sum LC omega-3 represents EPA+DPA+DHA. BMI, body mass index; DHA, docosapentaenoic acid; EPA, eicosapentaenoic acid; LC, long chain; NHANES, National Health and Nutrition Examination Survey.*"

The aim of their study was to determine reference ranges of circulating omega-3 PUFAs, EPA, DPA and DHA in a nationally representative population of Americans. Serum concentrations were compared with concentrations associated with consuming the recommended amount of EPA and DHA by the Dietary Guidelines for Americans and the Omega-3 Index (EPA + DHA). The setting was the National Health and Nutrition Examination Survey 2011–2012 cycle and the participants with fatty acids measured in serum were children aged 3–19 years and adults aged 20 years and older. The main measures were serum EPA, DPA, DHA and sum of omega-3 fatty acids expressed as percent of total fatty acids.

The findings, summarized in that table, are essentially that fatty acids concentrations in adults were found to be higher than that in children; more than 95% of children and 58% of adults had omega-3 concentrations below those recommended by Dietary Guidelines for Americans[*], and, not surprisingly, 89% of the adults had an Omega-3 Index in the "high cardiovascular risk" category. (19)

The need for criteria is both timely and pressing particularly in light of a study published in the journal *Nutrients*, in 2015, titled "Suboptimal Plasma Long Chain n-3 Concentrations Are Common among Adults in the United States, NHANES 2003–2004." The aim of the study was to describe plasma concentrations of omega-3 long-chain polyunsaturated fatty acids (n-3 LC-PUFA), mainly EPA (20:5 n-3) and DHA (22:6 n-3), and compare them to concentrations associated with cardiovascular health and dietary recommendations for two weekly servings of seafood.

Fasting plasma fatty acids were measured in participants 20 years old or older drawn from the National Health and Nutrition Examination Survey, 2003–2004. Fatty acids concentrations represent the sum of EPA, DHA and docosahexaenoic acid relative to total fatty acids (expressed as a percentage).

It was found that overall, 80.6% of participants had omega-3 LC-PUFA levels below concentrations recommended for cardiovascular health; nearly all participants (95.7%) had below-concentration levels associated with cardiovascular protection; participants 60 years or older had higher omega-3 PUFA concentrations than those aged 20–39 years but not those aged 40–59 years. Omega-3 PUFA concentrations were found to be lower in Hispanic participants relative to non-Hispanic black participants.

It was concluded that suboptimal long-chain omega-3 concentrations are common among US adults. And, the authors conclude that there is a need to increase intake among Americans. (20) And, by the way, the aforementioned *BMJ Open* study reported that approximately 89% of adults in their study had an Omega-3 Index in the high cardiovascular risk category.

It should be noted that, in addition to Omegaquant, there are a number of other "Omega-3 Index Home test" kits available online. Here is a sample of those:

- VitalChoice Omega-3 Index Home Test
- Dr. Guberman Omega-3 Index Plus Test

---

[*] The Dietary Guidelines for Americans provide nutritional advice for Americans who are healthy or who are at risk for chronic disease but do not currently have a chronic disease. The guidelines are published every five years by the US Department of Agriculture, together with the US Department of Health and Human Services. Notably, the most recent ninth edition for 2020–2025 includes dietary guidelines for children from birth to 23 months.

- Carlson Labs Omega-3 Test Kit
- Omega-3 Plus Patch

They range in price from $20.00 to $500.00 each.

Supplementing flaxseed or flaxseed oil seems to be a good avenue of achieving optimal omega-3 concentration given the published clinical evidence.

Disclaimer: First, we cannot vouch for the efficacy, reliability, validity or safety of any products that we cite as "examples." Second, we have no financial interest in any products that we cite as "examples."

9.3.1 Availability vs. Absorbability

It should be kept in mind that availability is not invariably absorbability. This is brought to our attention in a report in the *International Journal for Vitamin and Nutrition Research*, in 1998, titled "Can Adults Adequately Convert Alpha-Linolenic Acid (18:3n-3) to Eicosapentaenoic Acid (20:5n-3) and Docosahexaenoic acid (22:6n-3)?"

The author points out that a certain though restricted conversion of high doses of ALA to EPA occurs, but conversion to DHA is severely restricted. A background diet high in saturated fat restricts conversion to long-chain metabolites to approximately 6% for EPA and 3.8% for DHA. With a diet rich in omega-6 PUFA, conversion is nevertheless reduced by 40% to 50%.

The author further stipulates that we may need to focus on the adequate provision of DHA, which can reliably be achieved only with the supply of the preformed long-chain metabolite. (21) Similarly, guidelines for absorbability are also given in a report titled "Alpha-Linolenic Acid Supplementation and Conversion to n-3 Long-Chain Polyunsaturated Fatty Acids in Humans," published in the journal *Prostaglandins, Leukotrienes and Essential Fatty Acids* in 2009. (22)

9.4 ANTI-AGING ACTION OF L-ARGININE

"Anti-aging" is in quotes here because the term presents us with a conundrum: meant literally, one needs to be of advanced age to suffer from age-related diseases. But that is not what is commonly meant here. What we mean is that there are diseases that progress predictably as we age. This is the only meaning that validates the concept of anti-aging. Thus, anti-aging can be applied to the slowing or halting of the progression of what would otherwise be age-related diseases. In that sense, they are anti-aging, and they prolong life.

The amino acid L-arginine, plentiful in flaxseed, is said to be anti-aging. In previous chapters, it was noted that supplementation of flaxseed, therefore L-arginine, increased NO formation, the "Arginine Paradox"[*] notwithstanding. But as reported in many journal publications, enzymatic production of NO

---

[*] The Arginine Paradox: Exogenous L-arginine causes NO-mediated biological effects despite the fact that nitric oxide synthases (NOS) are theoretically saturated with L-arginine. (23)

declines steadily with increasing age, even in healthy people. Thus implementing strategies to diagnose and treat NO insufficiency may provide enormous benefits to the geriatric patient.

In a review published in the *Journal of Advanced Research* in 2010, titled "Anti-Aging Effects of L-Arginine," the author asserts that a number of clinical and experimental animal studies show that exogenous L-arginine intake is beneficial in doses larger than those in normal dietary consumption. Among the benefits cited is the reduction in the risk of vascular and heart diseases, reduction in erectile dysfunction, improvement in immune response and inhibition of gastric hyperacidity. Many, if not all, body functions are debilitated by aging. Studies have shown that L-arginine, through its versatile metabolic and physiological pathways, can improve many of these functions.

The author recites that arginine (1) increases the production of a variety of enzymes, hormones and structural proteins, (2) facilitates the release of growth hormone, insulin, glucagon and prolactin; (3) is involved in the action of vasopressin, produced by the pituitary gland; and (4) is a precursor of nitric oxide, polyamines, proline, glutamate, creatine, agmatine and urea. What's more, L-arginine boosts immunity, stimulates the thymus and promotes lymphocyte production, the key to promoting the healing of wounds and burns.

The author concludes from the review that *"the demonstrated anti-aging benefits of L-arginine show promises greater than any pharmaceutical or nutraceutical agent ever previously discovered."* (24)

The authors of a study titled "Endothelial Cellular Senescence Is Inhibited by Nitric Oxide: Implications in Atherosclerosis Associated with Menopause and Diabetes," published in the *Proceedings of the National Academy of Sciences USA*, in 2006, report investigating the effect of NO bioavailability on high glucose-promoted cellular senescence of umbilical vein endothelial cells.

They found that inhibition by eNOS transfection[*] of this cellular senescence under high glucose conditions was less pronounced. Treatment with L-arginine or L-citrulline of eNOS-transfected cells partially inhibited, and a combination of L-arginine and L-citrulline with antioxidants strongly prevented high glucose-induced cellular senescence. It was concluded that NO can prevent endothelial senescence, thereby contributing to the anti-senile action of estrogen. And, the ingestion of NO-boosting substances, including L-arginine, L-citrulline and antioxidants, can delay endothelial senescence under high glucose. (25)

The authors proposed that the delay in endothelial senescence through NO and/or eNOS activation may have clinical utility in the treatment of atherosclerosis in the elderly.

9.5 SUMMARY

Flaxseed and flax oil contain high amounts of omega-3 fatty acids. Clinical studies show that an ample supply of these constituents in body tissues slows cell aging

---

[*] Transfection is a procedure that introduces foreign nucleic acids into cells to produce genetically modified cells.

and reduces the risk of cardiovascular disease and premature death. There are now nonprescription blood tests, such as the Omegaquant Omega-3 Index, available to the public for assessing omega-3 body levels. Flaxseed also contains L-arginine, the precursor of nitric oxide that protects and enhances endothelial function.

9.6 REFERENCES

1. Harris WS, Mozaffarian D, Rimm E, Kris-Etherton P, Rudel LL, Appel LJ, Engler MM, Engler MB, and F Sacks. 2009. Omega-6 fatty acids and risk for cardiovascular disease. *Circulation*, 119: 902–907. DOI:10.1161/CIRCULATIONAHA.108.191627.
2. Harris WS. 2016. RBC omega-3 predicts risk for death. *Athersclerosis*, Sep 1; 252: P192–193. DOI:10.1016/j.atherosclerosis.2016.07.911.
3. www.cdc.gov/heartdisease/risk_factors.htm; accessed 17/12/21.
4. McBurney MI, Tintle NL, Vasan RS, Sala-Vila A, and WS Harris. 2021. Using an erythrocyte fatty acid fingerprint to predict risk of all-cause mortality: The Framingham Offspring Cohort. *American Journal of Clinical Nutrition*, Oct; 114(4): 1447–1454. DOI:10.1093/ajcn/nqab195.
5. Pottala JV, Garg S, Cohen BE, Whooley MA, and WS Harris. 2010. Blood eicosapentaenoic and docosahexaenoic acids predict all-cause mortality in patients with stable coronary heart disease: The heart and soul study. *Circulation: Cardiovascular Quality and Outcomes*, Jul; 3(4): 406–412. DOI:10.1161/CIRCOUTCOMES.109.896159.
6. Mozaffarian D, Lemaitre RN, King IB, Song X, Huang H, Sacks FM, Rimm EB, Wang M, and DS Siscovick. 2013. Plasma phospholipid long-chain ω-3 fatty acids and total and cause-specific mortality in older adults: A cohort study. *Annals of Internal Medicine*, Apr 2; 158(7): 515–525. DOI:10.7326/0003-4819-158-7-201304020-00003.
7. Harris WS, Tintle NL, Etherton MR, and RS Vasan. 2018. Erythrocyte long-chain omega-3 fatty acid levels are inversely associated with mortality and with incident cardiovascular disease: The framingham heart study. *Journal of Clinical Lipidology*, May–Jun; 12(3): 718–727.e6. DOI:10.1016/j.jacl.2018.02.010.
8. Harris WS, Luo J, Pottala JV, Espeland MAZ, Margolis KL, Manson JE, Wang L, Brasky TM, and JG Robinson. 2017. Red blood cell polyunsaturated fatty acids and mortality in the Women's Health Initiative Memory Study. *Journal of Clinical Lipidology*, Jan–Feb; 11(1): 250–259.e5. DOI:10.1016/j.jacl.2016.12.013.
9. Kleber ME, Delgado GE, Lorkowski S, März W, and C von Schacky. 2016. Omega-3 fatty acids and mortality in patients referred for coronary angiography. The ludwigshafen risk and cardiovascular health study. *Atherosclerosis*, Sep; 252: 175–181. DOI:10.1016/j.atherosclerosis.2016.06.049.
10. Kiecolt-Glaser JK, Epel ES, Belury MA, Andridge R, Lin J, Glaser R, Malarkey WB, Hwang BS, and E Blackburne. 2013. Omega-3 fatty acids, oxidative stress, and leukocyte telomere length: A randomized controlled trial. *Brain, Behavior and Immunity*, Feb; 28: 16–24. DOI:10.1016/j.bbi.2012.09.004.
11. Dixon JA, and FG Spinale. 2011. Myocardial remodeling: Cellular and extracellular events and targets. *Annual Review of Physiology*, Mar 17; 73: 47–68. DOI:10.1146/annurev-physiol-012110-142230.
12. Pepe S. 2005. Effect of dietary polyunsaturated fatty acids on age-related changes in cardiac mitochondrial membranes. *Experimental Gerontology*, Aug–Sep; 40(8–9): 751–758. DOI:10.1016/j.exger.2005.03.013.
13. Lalia AZ, Dasari S, Robinson MM, Abid H, Morse DM, Klaus KA, and IR Lanza. 2017. Influence of omega-3 fatty acids on skeletal muscle protein metabolism and mitochondrial

bioenergetics in older adults. *Aging* (Albany NY), Apr; 9(4): 1096–1129. DOI:10.18632/aging.101210.
14. Afshordel S, Hagl S, Werner D, Röhner N, Kögel D, Bazan NG, and GP Eckert. 2015. Omega-3 polyunsaturated fatty acids improve mitochondrial dysfunction in brain aging—impact of Bcl-2 and NPD-1 like metabolites. *Prostaglandins, Leukotrienes and Essential Fatty Acids*, Jan; 92: 23–31. DOI:10.1016/j.plefa.2014.05.008.
15. Denis I, Potier B, Vancassel S, Heberden C, and M Lavialle. 2013. Omega-3 fatty acids and brain resistance to ageing and stress: Body of evidence and possible mechanisms. *Ageing Research Reviews*, Mar; 12(2): 579–594. DOI:10.1016/j.arr.2013.01.007.
16. Zamroziewicz MK, Paul EJ, Zwilling CE, and AK Barbey. 2018. Determinants of fluid intelligence in healthy aging: Omega-3 polyunsaturated fatty acid status and frontoparietal cortex structure. *Nutritional Neuroscience*, 21(8): 570–579. DOI:10.1080/1028415X.2017.1324357.
17. Gupta R, Dhatwalia S, Chaudhry M, Kondal D, Stein AD, Prabhakaran D, Tandon N, Ramakrishnan L, and S Khandelwa. 2021. Standardization and validation of assay of selected omega-3 and omega-6 fatty acids from phospholipid fraction of red cell membrane using gas chromatography with flame ionization detector. *Journal of Analytical Science and Technology*, Aug; 12(1): 33. DOI:10.1186/s40543-021-00287-1.
18. Harris WS. 2008. The omega-3 index as a risk factor for coronary heart disease. *American Journal of Clinical Nutrition*, Jun; 87(6): 1997S–2002S. DOI:10.1093/ajcn/87.6.1997S.
19. Murphy RA, Devarshi PP, Ekimura S, Marshall K, and SH Mitmesser. 2021. Long-chain omega-3 fatty acid serum concentrations across life stages in the USA: An analysis of NHANES 2011–2012. *BMJ Open*, 11: e043301. DOI:10.1136/bmjopen-2020-043301.
20. Murphy RA, Yu EA, Ciappio ED, Mehta S, and MI McBurney. 2015. Suboptimal plasma long chain n-3 concentrations are common among adults in the United States, NHANES 2003–2004. *Nutrients*, Dec 9; 7(12): 10282–10289. DOI:10.3390/nu7125534.
21. Gerster H. 1998. Can adults adequately convert alpha-linolenic acid (18:3n-3) to eicosapentaenoic acid (20:5n-3) and docosahexaenoic acid (22:6n-3)? *International Journal for Vitamin and Nutrition Research*, 68(3): 159–173. PMID: 9637947.
22. Brenna JT, Salem N Jr, Sinclair AJ, Cunnane SC, and International Society for the Study of Fatty Acids and Lipids, ISSFAL. 2009. Alpha-Linolenic acid supplementation and conversion to n-3 long-chain polyunsaturated fatty acids in humans. *Prostaglandins, Leukotrienes and Essential Fatty Acids*, Feb–Mar; 80(2–3): 85–91. DOI:10.1016/j.plefa.2009.01.004.
23. Nakaki T, and K Hishikawa. 2002. The arginine paradox [Article in Japanese]. *Nihon Yakurigaku Zasshi* [Folia Pharmacologica Japonica], Jan; 119(1): 7–14. DOI:10.1254/fpj.119.7.
24. Gad MZ. 2010. Anti-aging effects of l-arginine. *Journal of Advanced Research*, Jul; 1(3): 169–177. DOI:10.1016/j.jare.2010.05.001.
25. Hayashi T, Matsui-Hirai H, Miyazaki-Akita A, Fukatsu A, Funami J, Ding Q-F, Kamalanathan S, Hattori Y, Ignarro LJ, and A Iguchi. 2006. Endothelial cellular senescence is inhibited by nitric oxide: Implications in atherosclerosis associated with menopause and diabetes. *Proceedings of the National Academy of Sciences USA*, Nov 7; 103(45): 17018–17023. DOI:10.1073/pnas.0607873103.
26. Harman D. 1956. Aging: A theory based on free radical and radiation chemistry. *Journal of Gerontology*, Jul; 11(3): 298–300. DOI:10.1093/geronj/11.3.298.
27. Harris WS, and C Von Schacky. 2004. The Omega-3 Index: A new risk factor for death from coronary heart disease? *Preventive Medicine*, Jul; 39(1): 212–220. DOI:10.1016/j.ypmed.2004.02.030.

Index

Note: Page numbers in *italics* indicate a figure and page numbers in **bold** indicate a table on the corresponding page.

A

acetylcholine (ACh), 7, 31–32, 49, 154–155
adjuvant treatment of type 2 diabetes, flaxseed in, 129–138, *see also* type 2 diabetes
    treatment dosage matters, 134
    L-arginine as, 134–138
ad lib supplementation, 18–22
    flax oil, 18–19
    golden flaxseed vs. brown flaxseed, 19–20
    ground flaxseeds, 18
    macronutrients, 19
    raw flaxseed, 19–20
    whole flaxseeds, 18
aging effect, in erectile dysfunction (ED), 159–162
alanine aminotransferase (ALT), 139
albuginea, 159
albumin-creatinine ratio (ACR), 140
alpha-linoleic acid (ALA), 4–5, 8, 11–14, 20, 25, 70, 93, 129, 151
    content of selected foods, 12, **13**
    in eNO formation, 70–71
alpha-linolenic acid/low fat (ALF), 70, 73
American Heart Association (AHA), 6, 32, 109
amino acid L-arginine, 8
amino acids, 27
1-amino D-proline (1ADP), 38
aminotransferase (AST), 139
amygdalin, 3, 53
anti-aging action of L-arginine, 178–179
anticoagulant drugs, 36
antidiabetic benefit, 38, **39**
antifungal benefit, 38, **39**
antihypertensive benefit, 38, **39**
anti-nutritional aspects of flaxseed, 37–38
    CNglcs, 34–35
    hydrogen cyanide, 37
    linamarin, 35
    neolinustatin, 37
    phytic acid, 38
antioxidants, 19, 38, **39**
anti-platelet drugs, 36
anti-thrombic benefit, 38, **39**
anti-tumor benefit, 38, **39**
arginine paradox, 118, 143
arterial vessel compliance, 72–74
arterial waveform, 74–76
    diastolic phase, 75
    dicrotic notch, 75
    systolic phase, 75
asymmetric dimethyl L-arginine (ADMA), 78, 83, 117
    Arginine Paradox and, 118
    as L-arginine's analogue, 117–118
atherosclerosis, 49, 89–104
    atherosclerotic plaque, 89, *90*
    endothelial glycocalyx in, 60
    L-arginine in preventing/reversing, 97–99
    omega-3 fatty acids and NO from flax intervention in, 89–104
    polyunsaturated fatty acids (PUFAs) in preventing/reversing, 93
    rheumatoid arthritis, 102–103
    ROS role in, 92

B

benign prostate hypertrophy (BPH), 153
blood flow control systems, 80
blood platelets, 33
blood pressure
    drugs, 36
    endothelium-dependent control of, 79–80
    endothelium-independent control of, 79
    eNO in controlling, 79–83
    L-arginine supplementation reducing, 114–117
    reduction, by flax/omega-3 fatty acids, 111–113
    treatment, 10
blood through the circulatory system, 68–71
blood urea nitrogen (BUN), 139
blood vessel and heart function, 67–85
    arterial vessel compliance, 72–74
    arterial waveform, 74–76
    flaxseed micronutrients role in, 67–85
    nitric oxide (NO) role in, 67–85
    peripheral artery disease (PAD) combating, 83–85
blood vessels (*Vasa Vasorum*), 54–56
    depends on endothelium derived NO vasorelaxation, 56
    NO regulating, 54–56
    structure and function of, 55–56
bread recipe, 21
brown flaxseed, 19–20

183

C

canola oil (CanO), 145
cardiovascular disease (CVD), 10, 155, 170
Carlson Labs Omega-3 test kit, 178
catalase (CAT), 126
cellulose, 28
cholesterol esters (CEs), 101
cholesterol-lowering benefit of flax proteins, 38, **39**
chronic heart failure, 144–145
chronic kidney disease (CKD), 34, 138–145
    flax, inflammation, and endothelium dysfunction in, 138–145
    flaxseed as adjuvant treatment of, 138–139
    hypertension and chronic heart failure and, 144–145
    L-arginine in treatment of, 142–144
    omega-3 fatty acids in adjuvant treatment of, 14, 139–142
chronic renal failure (CRF) treatment, L-arginine in, 16
chronic systemic inflammation (CSI), 99–103
    C-reactive protein (CRP) in, 99
    L-arginine reducing, 102
    omega-3 ALA reducing, 101–102
    omega-3 fatty acids intervention in, 89–104
Cialis®, 153
cognitive aging, 174–175
common flax (*Linum usitatissimum* L.), 1
conditional amino acids, 27
constitutive nitric oxide synthase (cNOS), 51–52
Cool Knight brand grinder, 37
coronary heart disease, 9, 132
    omega-3 PUFAs in treatment of, 12
    type 2 diabetes and, 132
corpora cavernosae, 158, *158*
corpora spongeosum, 158, *158*
C-reactive protein (CRP), 99–103
creatinine clearance (Ccr), 144–145
cross-check dietary history method, 127
Cuisinart brand grinder, 37
cyanogenic glycosides (CNglcs) in flaxseeds, 3–4, 6, 8, 34–35, 99, 113, 125, 151
cyclic guanosine monophosphate (cGMP), 53, 159
cyclosporin A (CYS), 139

D

daily diet, flaxseed in, 21–22
diabetes, *see also* type 2 diabetes
    drugs, 36
    endothelial glycocalyx in, 59–60
diabetic nephropathy, type 2 diabetes with, 133–134
diastolic phase, 75
dicrotic notch, 75
Dietary Approaches to Stop Hypertension (DASH), 115
dietary fiber, 28–29
digital-subtracted arteriography, 114
dihydrotestosterone (DHT), 153
dimethylarginine dimethylaminohydrolase (DDAH), 118
docosahexaenoic acid (DHA), 8, 11–14, 12, **13**, 25, 93–94, 102, 112–113, 131, 170, 175
Dr. Guberman Omega-3 index plus test, 177
dyslipidemia treatment, 9

E

eicosapentaenoic acid (EPA), 8, 11–14, 12, **13**, 25, 93–94, 102, 112, 131, 170, 175
ejection fraction, 71
endocardium, 69
endothelial dysfunction
    in L-arginine therapy, 119–120
    in sickle cell disease therapy, 119–120
    treatment, L-arginine in, 15
    treatment, omega-3 PUFAs in, 12
    in type 2 diabetes, 128
endothelial glycocalyx, 56–59
    in atherosclerosis, 60
    in diabetes, 59–60
    glycocalyx regulate eNO formation, 58–59
    in health and disease, 59–61
    in hypertension, 60–61
endothelial nitric oxide (eNO) bioavailability, 14, 45–62, 81, 151, 156–157
    in blood pressure control, 79–83
    blood vessels regulated by NO, 54–56
    endothelial glycocalyx, 56–59
    endothelial NO from L-Arginine, 51–52
    endothelium, 47–49
    formation, 52–53
    L-arginine beneficial effect on, 45–62
    NO from CNglcs, 53–54
    omega-3 PUFA beneficial effect on, 45–62
    oxidative stress in endothelium damage, 50–51
    reactive oxygen species (ROS) in endothelium damage, 50–51
endothelial nitric oxide synthase (eNOS), 51–52, 81
endothelium, structure and function of, 47–49, 154
endothelium-derived relaxing factor (EDRF), 49, 154
endothelium dysfunction, erectile dysfunction (ED) and, 162
enterodiol (ED), 95
epinephrine, 79

Index

erectile dysfunction (ED), 50, 153
  aging role in, 159–162
  causes of, 153–154
  endothelium dysfunction as a feature of, 162
  flaxseed in, 162–165
  L-arginine in treating, 16, 163
  omega-3 fatty acids in treating, 164–165
  reactive oxygen species (ROS) jeopardizing, 155–156
  sexual performance and, 161–162
erythrocyte deformability, 33
essential amino acids, 27
essential fats, 20
estimated glomerular filtration rate (eGFR), 133

F

fat mass (FM), 135
fatty acids profile in flaxseed oil, 26–27, **27**
Finasteride (Propecia®), 153
Flax Council of Canada, 4
flax fibers, 28
flax/flax plant
  bleeding chances increased, 7
  in blood pressure lowering, 7
  in blood sugar lowering, 7
  consumption, safety, 3–6
  as a functional food, 2–3
  in garment of pharaohs, 1–2
  health uses, 1–2
  on hormones, 7
  supplement dosages, 7–18
  uses, 1–2
flaxseed, 8–11
  as adjuvant treatment of CKD, 138–139
  as adjuvant treatment of type 2 diabetes, 129–138
  in blood pressure reduction, 10, 111–113
  in cardiovascular risk factors prevention, 10
  CNglcs safety in, 113
  constituents contribution in type 2 diabetes, 125–128
  in coronary artery disease treatment, 9
  dosages, 8–9
  dyslipidemia, 9
  in erectile dysfunction (ED) treatment, 162–165
  in hypertension treatment, 9, 109–120
  flow-mediated dilation (FMD) improved by, 77–78
  in metabolic syndrome treatment, 9–10
  micronutrients, in blood vessel and heart function, 67–85
  in obesity and insulin resistance treatment, 10
  oil, 18–19, 26–27
  type 2 diabetes, 10

flow-mediated dilation (FMD), 60, 76–78, 116
  flaxseed improving, 77–78
  L-arginine improving, 77–78
  measuring blood flow by, 76–78
foam cells, 56
Food and Drug Administration (FDA), 3
free-fat mass (FFM), 135
functional food, flaxseed as, 2–3, 25–39
  constituents, 25–26
  dietary fiber, 28–29
  fatty acids profile in flaxseed oil, 26–27, **27**
  flaxseed oil/lipids components, 26–27
  health benefits, 25–39
  lignans, 29
  minerals, 29
  nutrient and phytochemicals, composition, 26, **26**
  proteins, 27–28

G

gamma-glutamyltransferase (GGT), 133
gas fuels performance, 154–155
β-gentiobioside of acetone cyanohydrin, 34–35
glomerular filtration rate (GFR), 140
glucose-stimulated insulin secretion (GSIS), 137
glycocalyx, 157
  eNO formation regulation, 58–59
  glycocalyx/eSL (endothelial surface layer), 56
goitrogens, 4–5
golden flaxseed, 19–20
Greek Mediterranean diet, 111
ground flaxseeds, 18
guanosine triphosphate (GTP), 53
guanylyl cyclase, 53

H

Harman theory, 172
health benefits of flaxseed, 29–34
  acetylcholine (Ach) production increase, 31–32
  benign prostate hypertrophy risk lowering, 33
  blood glucose level reduction, 33
  blood pressure decrease, 32
  blood viscosity decrease, 32–33
  cardiac arrest risk reduction, 32
  cardiovascular disease prevention, 32
  flax proteins, 38–39
  health hazards of menopause improvement, 34
  healthy bowel function promotion, 33
  heart arrhythmias incidence reduction, 32
  heart function improvement, 32
  heart muscle lipid fluidity increase, 32
  insulin production increase, 33
  joint pain and arthritis reduction, 33
  kidney function improvement, 34
  lipid profile improvement, 34

liver function improvement, 34
proinflammatory cytokines level decrease, 30
serotonin production increase, 30–31
health span
   cognitive aging, 174–175
   L-arginine increasing, 169–180
   omega-3 PUFA increasing, 169–180
health targets of functional elements of flaxseed, 30, *31*
heart disease, 155
   treatment, L-arginine in, 15
   treatment, omega-3 PUFAs in, 12
heart function, 67–85
   chambers and valves, 68, *69*
   systole, 68–70
hematocrit, 33
hemodialysis (HD), 100, 145
high-density lipoprotein (HDL), 94
high-sensitivity C-reactive protein (hs-CRP) test, 77
HOMA-IR index, 130
homeostasis model assessment (HOMA-IR), 133
hydrogen cyanide, 37
hypertension, 109–120, 144–145
   endothelial glycocalyx in, 60–61
   flaxseed combating, 82–83
   flaxseed in treatment of, 109–120
   L-arginine in treatment of, 109–120
   as omega-3 deficiency, 110–111
   omega-3 fatty acids in treatment of, 109–120
   reduction, by flax/omega-3 fatty acids, 111–113
   treatment, 9
hypocaloric diet, 135

I

icosapent ethyl, 14
inducible nitric oxide synthase (iNOS), 51–52
inositol triphosphate (IP3), 52
insulin resistance, omega-3 fatty acids reducing, 131
interleukin 6, 78
intermittent claudication, L-arginine in, 16
International Index of Erectile Function (IIEF) score, 163
isoproterenol (isuprel), 17

K

kidney function, omega-3 PUFAs in, 14, *see also* chronic kidney disease

L

L-arginine (Arg), 3, 7, 14–18
   anti-aging action of, 178–179
   asymmetric dimethylarginine (ADMA) as an analogue of, 117
   in atherosclerosis prevention/reversing, 93
   beneficial effect on eNO, 45–62
   in chronic kidney disease treatment, 142–144
   in chronic renal failure (CRF) treatment, 16
   in chronic systemic inflammation (CSI) reduction, 102
   dosage recommendations, 15
   in endothelial dysfunction treatment, 15, 119–120
   in erectile dysfunction (ED) treatment, 16–17, 163
   flow-mediated dilation (FMD) improved by, 77–78
   health span increase by, 169–180
   in heart disease treatment, 15
   in hypertension treatment 109–120
   intermittent claudication treatment, 16
   life span increase by, 169–180
   in myocardial infarction treatment, 16
   in peripheral artery disease (PAD) treatment, 16
   in sickle cell disease treatment, 16
   supplementation, in blood pressure reduction, 114–117
   in type 2 diabetes treatment, 17, 125–146
lariciresinol, 29
life span
   availability vs. absorbability, 178
   cognitive aging, 174–175
   flaxseed consumers, 171–175
   L-arginine increasing, 169–180
   omega-3 PUFA increasing, 169–180
   preventing the shortening of, 169–171
lignans, 29
linamarin, 35, 53
linatine, 38
linen textiles from flax, 2
linoleic acid, 20
linustatin, 4, 34–35, 53
lipid peroxidation (LPO), 126
loaf recipe, 21
lower urinary tract symptoms (LUTS), 33
lumen, 157
lutein, 19

M

macronutrients, 19
malondialdehyde (MDA), 74, 126
matairesinol, 29
metabolic syndrome treatment, 9–10, 14
methyl ethyl ketone cyanohydrins, 35
Michaelis-Menten constant (Km), 118
micronutrients, 2
mitochondria free radical "emissions," 172–174

Index

Molecule of the Year, 1992, 46, *see* nitric oxide
mononuclear cells (MNCs), 95
5-monophosphate (cGMP), 144
MotorGenic brand grinder, 37
mucilage gums, 28
muffins recipe, 21
myocardial infarction treatment, L-arginine in, 16

N

neolinustatin, 4, 34–35, 37, 53
neurotransmitters, 47, 154
nicotinamide adenine dinucleotide phosphate (NADPH), 92
nitrates, 17
nitric oxide (NO), 7–8, 45–46, 151; *see also* sexual function
    in atherosclerosis, 89–104
    bioavailability, flaxseed increasing, 70
    in blood vessel and heart function, 67–85
    in chronic systemic inflammation, 89–104
    from CNglcs, 53–54
    from flaxseed enhancing sexual function, 151–166
    formation in body, 49–50
nitric oxide synthases (NOS), 7, 97, 137
nonalcoholic fatty liver disease (NAFLD), 34, 132–133
nonessential amino acids, 27
norepinephrine, 79
nutraceuticals, 3

O

obesity and insulin resistance treatment, 10
oleic/low fat (OLF), 73
omega-3 ALA, in CSI reduction, 101–102
omega-3 fatty acids, 70–71, 111–113
    in adjuvant treatment of kidney disease, 139–142
    as adjuvant treatment of NAFLD, 132–133
    in atherosclerosis, 89–104
    blood pressure reduction by, 111–113
    in chronic kidney disease treatment, 125–146
    in chronic systemic inflammation, 89–104
    from elevated blood cholesterol, 94–96
    in eNO formation, 70–71
    in erectile dysfunction (ED) treatment, 164–165
    from flaxseed, 93–94, 96–97
    in hypertension treatment, 109–120
    insulin resistance reduction by, 131
    in triglycerides reduction in Type 2 diabetes, 131–132
    in type 2 diabetes treatment, 125–146

Omega-3 Index, 111–113, 131, 175–178
Omega-3 Index Home test, 177
Omega-3 plus patch, 178
omega-3 polyunsaturated fatty acids (PUFAs), 3, 11–14
    aging slowed down by, 172–174
    cell aging and, 171–172
    in chronic kidney disease (CKD) treatment, 14
    content of selected foods, 12, **13**
    in coronary heart disease treatment, 12
    in endothelial dysfunction treatment, 12
    eNO effect on, 45–62
    health span increase by, 169–180
    in heart disease treatment, 12
    icosapent ethyl, 14
    intake of, 11, **11**
    in kidney function and myocardial infarction treatment, 14
    life span increase by, 169–180
    in metabolic syndrome treatment, 14
    in type 2 diabetes treatment, 13
omega-3-acid ethyl esters, 14
omega-3-carboxylic acids, 14
oral drugs, 36
oral glucose tolerance test, 127
oxidative stress, 155–156
    in endothelium damage, 50–51
    in type 2 diabetes, 126–127

P

p-coumaric acid, 29
penis, 158–159, *see also* sexual function
corpora cavernosae, 158
    corpora spongeosum, 158
    cross-section of, 158, *158*
    penile erection, ACH/NO/CGMP pathway to, 159
Perfumed Garden of the Shaykh Nefzawi, The, 152
peripheral artery disease (PAD)
    flaxseed combating, 83–85
    treatment, 16
phosphodiesterase (PDE), 53
phosphodiesterase type-5 (PDE5), 159
phospholipids, 101
phytic acid, 5, 38
pinoresinol, 29
placebo effect, 151
plasma viscosity, 32–33
polyphenol, 19
polyunsaturated fatty acids (PUFAs), 93
Prima Cucina brand grinder, 37
proteins, 27–28
prunasin, 53
pyridoxal 5′-phosphate (P-5-P), 38

Q

QUICKI index, 130

R

raw flaxseed, 19–20
reactive oxygen species (ROS), 91, 151, 155–156
   in atherosclerosis, 91
   in endothelium damage, 50–51
   jeopardizing erectile function, 155–156
red blood cell (erythrocyte) deformability, 33
renin-angiotensin-aldosterone system (RAAS), 60–61
rheumatoid arthritis, 102–103

S

S-adenosylmethionine, 118
saturated fatty acids (SFAs), 165
saturated/high fat (SHF), 73
secoisolariciresinol (SECO), 95
secoisolariciresinol diglucoside (SDG), 29, 34, 67, 71, 95
SELFNutritionData, 35
serum creatinine (Cr), 145
sexual desire vs. sexual performance, 151–152
sexual function, 151–166, *see also* erectile dysfunction; penis
   gas fuels performance, 154–155
   NO from flaxseed enhancing, 151–166
   oyster and the blue pill, 151–152
   penis, 158–159
   Perfumed Garden of the Shaykh Nefzawi, The, 152
   as shunting blood flow in the body, 157–159
shunting blood flow in the body, 157–159
sickle cell disease (SCD), 109–120
   endothelial dysfunction in, 119–120
   flaxseed in treatment of, 109–120
   L-arginine in treatment of, 16, 109–120
   omega-3 fatty acids in treatment of, 109–120
signal molecule, 47
Sildenafil (Viagra), 17
snack recipe, 21
superoxide dismutase (SOD), 58, 126
supplementation, flaxseed, 7–18
   ALA, recommended content, 37
   in clinical and research trials, 7–18
   guidelines, 35–37
   interactions involved, 36
systole, 68–70, 75

T

testosterone, 151
thiocyanates, 4
tortillas recipe, 21
total cholesterol (TC), 94
triglycerides (TG), 95, 98
tumor necrosis factor-α (TNF-α), 77–78
tunica, 159
Turimon brand grinder, 37
type 2 diabetes, 125–146
   coronary heart disease and, 132
   endothelial dysfunction in, 128
   flaxseed as adjuvant treatment of, 129–138
   flaxseed constituents contribution in, 125–128
   L-arginine in treatment of, 125–146
   no deficiency disease, question of, 134–138
   omega-3 fatty acids in treatment of, 125–146
   omega-3 fatty acids reduce triglycerides in, 131–132
   oxidative stress in, 126–127
   treatment, L-arginine in, 17
   treatment, omega-3 PUFAs in, 13

U

uric acid (UA), 139
urinary sodium excretion rate (UNa), 144

V

vagus material, 49
vascular remodeling in hypertension, 80–82
vasculogenic erectile dysfunction (VED), 164
Viagra® (Sildenafil), 53, 153, 159

W

Western(ized) Diet, 114
whole flaxseeds 18, 28

Z

zeaxanthin, 19